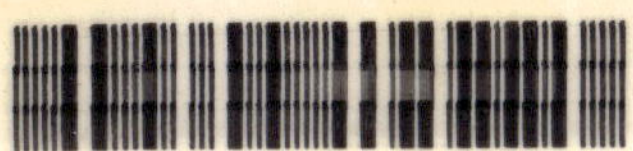

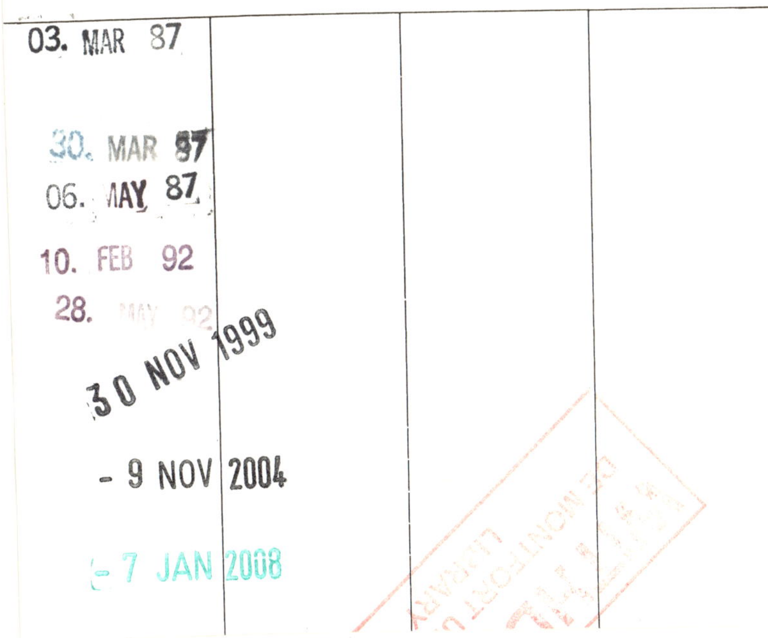

Monographs on Endocrinology

Volume 6

Edited by

F. Gross, Heidelberg · A. Labhart, Zürich

T. Mann, Cambridge · L. T. Samuels, Salt Lake City

J. Zander, München

K. Federlin

Immunopathology of Insulin

Clinical and Experimental Studies

With 53 Figures

1971
William Heinemann Medical Books Ltd., London
Springer-Verlag Berlin · Heidelberg · New York

Privatdozent Dr. KONRAD FEDERLIN
Wissenschaftlicher Rat

Universität Ulm
Medizinisch-Naturwissenschaftliche Hochschule
Zentrum für Innere Medizin und Kinderheilkunde
Ulm/Donau

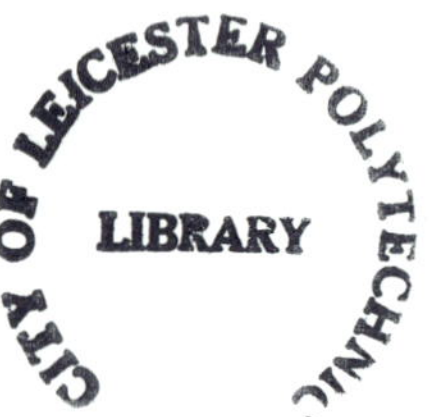

ISBN 0-433-10310-8 William Heinemann Medical Books Ltd. London
ISBN 3-540-05408-1 Springer-Verlag Berlin Heidelberg New York
ISBN 0-387-05408-1 Springer-Verlag New York Heidelberg Berlin

Printed in Germany. Type-setting, printing and binding: Konrad Triltsch, Graphischer Betrieb, 87 Würzburg, Germany

Dedicated
to
my wife and my children

Preface

Soon after the discovery of insulin in 1922, it became clear that the use of this hormone in the treatment of diabetics is often accompanied by allergy. In 1956 it became possible to determine quantitatively the insulin-binding antibodies which are responsible for the resistance to insulin. The methods developed since then make it possible to measure minute amounts of the pancreatic hormone in blood and extracellular fluids.

There have been many attempts to relate insulin allergy and insulin resistance to the primary, secondary or tertiary structure of the A or B chains, or both, and more recently, to the proinsulin which is present in all commercial preparations of insulin, i. e. to the species-specific structure of the C peptide. In the great majority of papers dealing either with the immunogenic and antigenic properties of insulin or with the relevant antibodies, the discussion has been restricted to the humoral antibodies. The existence of a brief period of delayed local allergy resulting from the cellular immune response has more or less escaped attention.

It is specifically this period of delayed allergy that attracted the interest of Dr. FEDERLIN and his colleagues. Making use of immunohistological and other techniques which are rarely employed in clinical observation, and with the help of experiments on animals, Dr. FEDERLIN traces the course of insulin allergy from cellular immunity, through the production of humoral antibodies by the insulin-binding cells of the circulation, to the sessile immunological apparatus.

It remains to be seen whether the problems of insulin allergy can be resolved by improvements in the preparation of insulin, involving either the synthesis of human insulin or further purification of the hormone from animal material. In the meantime, this monograph provides a convincing demonstration of the value of clinical observations when these are reinforced by modern laboratory techniques. Dr. FEDERLIN is to be congratulated on a brilliant contribution to a problem which is of interest to endocrinologists and diabetologists alike, as well as to immunologists.

Ulm, April 1971

E. F. PFEIFFER

Contents

A. Introduction

Following the discovery of insulin in 1922 and the institution of the treatment of diabetes mellitus with extracts of animal pancreas, the immunological side-effects of this therapy came under consideration. While insulin allergy causes problems at the very beginning of therapy with insulin, what complicates long-term therapy is resistance to insulin. Both types of immune reaction are consequent upon the immunogenicity of insulin (or injected extracts of pancreatic tissue). Insulin-neutralizing antibodies have long been the object of numerous investigations by a variety of techniques. Interest in the localized allergic reaction was limited, until recently. This lack of scientific interest is perhaps to be explained by the transience of the local reaction; thus there are few systematic investigations of the origin of this frequent side effect. The basis of the present investigation is mainly clinical experience in a large out-patient department for diabetics at the First University Medical Clinic, Frankfurt am Main, and, in part, also the out-patient service for diabetics at the Center for Internal Medicine, University of Ulm. Thorough questioning of diabetic patients who had recently started insulin therapy disclosed that localized inflammatory reactions occur extremely often, but are not reported to the doctor because they recede spontaneously in a few days. A review of the literature affords no unified concept of the nature and course of these allergic reactions. Since all insulin-treated diabetics show insulin-binding antibodies in the serum after a few months, the assumption is that the delayed-onset, localized skin reaction represents a stage of delayed hypersensitivity to insulin — a "normal" consequence of the repeated parenteral injection of foreign proteins. The present studies of diabetic subjects are concerned principally with this problem. Since this phenomenon cannot be evaluated apart from humoral antibodies to insulin, these too were investigated although not to the same extent. Systematic clinical and laboratory investigations of patients have their intrinsic limitations; therefore it was decided to study the course of immune reactions after injection of insulin in animal experiments as well. Thus, out of one clinical observation there arose a complex of related studies, extending over a period of several years, on the immunopathology of insulin. Great parts of these studies would not have been possible without the untiring assistance of my coworker, Dr. G. HEINEMANN, and the skilful technical assistance of Mrs. E. ESPINOZA, to whom I am especially grateful. Furthermore I am much indebted for additional help to Drs. D. KRIEGBAUM, F. SORGE, I. GIGLI, B. BECKER, M. BIEDERMANN and to Miss M. SCHÄFER.

Finally I wish to express my thanks to the Head of the Department of Endocrinology and Metabolism, Professor E. F. PFEIFFER, for his constant support, criticism and encouragement during all the years of work.

B. Brief Review of the Immunology of Insulin

I. Antigenicity of Insulin

For a long time, no antigenic properties were attributed to insulin. Up to the present, it remains controversial whether insulin is a weak or a strong antigen. On the one hand, hormones were not regarded as antigens due to their species-unspecific biological activity, while on the other hand, insulin is a very small molecule in comparison with other proteins. Indeed, LEWIS (1937) was able to demonstrate that guinea-pig uterus, immunized with bovine or porcine insulin, reacted by contracting in the presence of the antigen (SCHULTZ-DALE technique). HAUROWITZ (1950), however, still considered the antigenic property of insulin quite improbable.

Greater insight was achieved with the determination of the chemical structure of different insulins by SANGER (1960). In its monomeric form this hormone has a molecular weight of approximately 6000, but it exists mostly as a polymer whose size depends on such factors as the pH of the solution, ionic strength, etc. (ONCLEY et al., 1952). The molecule consists of two polypeptide chains, an A-chain with 21 amino acids and a B-chain with 30. Both chains are bound to each other at the cystine site by two disulfide bridges (Fig. 1 a). Those mammalian insulins whose structure has been determined, up to the present, demonstrate that the molecules differ in the amino acids at positions 8,9 and 10 of the A-chains (HARRIS, SANGER and NAUGHTON, 1956; BEHRENS and BROMER, 1958; ISHIHARA et al., 1958; SANGER, 1959). But human insulin differs in that it contains an alanine-substituted threonine in position 30 of the B-chain (NICOL and SMITH, 1960).

At first it was assumed that the antigenic determinants were localized solely in these molecular regions, and that most of the insulin could be regarded as immunologically indifferent (BURNET, 1961). Meanwhile it began to appear that conditions were really more complicated than that. Thus BERSON and YALOW (1963) showed that porcine insulin, which differs from human insulin only in the terminal amino acid of the B-chain (alanine instead of threonine), affected antibody formation in diabetics even when this terminal amino acid — itself the antigen-determining group — was separated from the molecule.

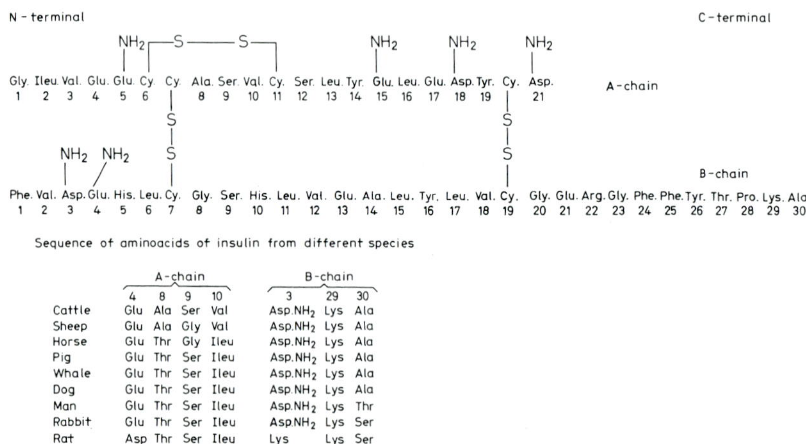

Sequence of aminoacids of insulin from different species

	A-chain				B-chain		
	4	8	9	10	3	29	30
Cattle	Glu	Ala	Ser	Val	Asp.NH2	Lys	Ala
Sheep	Glu	Ala	Gly	Val	Asp.NH2	Lys	Ala
Horse	Glu	Thr	Gly	Ileu	Asp.NH2	Lys	Ala
Pig	Glu	Thr	Ser	Ileu	Asp.NH2	Lys	Ala
Whale	Glu	Thr	Ser	Ileu	Asp.NH2	Lys	Ala
Dog	Glu	Thr	Ser	Ileu	Asp.NH2	Lys	Ala
Man	Glu	Thr	Ser	Ileu	Asp.NH2	Lys	Thr
Rabbit	Glu	Thr	Ser	Ileu	Asp.NH2	Lys	Ser
Rat	Asp	Thr	Ser	Ileu	Lys	Lys	Ser

Fig. 1 a. Sequence of amino acids of insulin from different species

During recent years the explanation for this was sought in differences of the spatial configuration which is still unknown, although some hypotheses have been proposed (LINDERSTRÖM-LANG, 1955; LINDLAY and ROLLETT, 1955; LOW and EDSALL, 1956; ARQUILLA, BROMER and MERCOLA, 1969). ARQUILLA et al. presented evidence that the C-terminal A-chain and C-terminal B-chain in close proximity to each other form a center rich in aromatic amino acids. (Figs. 1 a and 1 b).

This center seemed to be important, not only for the conformation of antigenic determinants, but also for the biologic effect of the molecule. Insulin derivatives with greater distortion of antigenic determinants (desoctapeptid, iodinated, triconjugated fluorescein insulin) also showed negligible biological insulin activity. Change in conformation results in a proportional decrease in biologic activity. Using synthetic polypeptides WILSON (1969) demonstrated that guinea pig antibodies to bovine insulin reacted with determinants within the regions A_{10-16}, B_{1-8}, B_{24-30}.

An unexpected antigenicity of insulin was demonstrated in cattle and sheep (RENOLD, SOELDNER and STEINKE, 1964; RENOLD et al., 1965). Subcutaneous injections of homologous insulin produced antibody response and severe lesions of the islets of Langerhans, i. e. autoaggression occurred.

BOVINE INSULIN

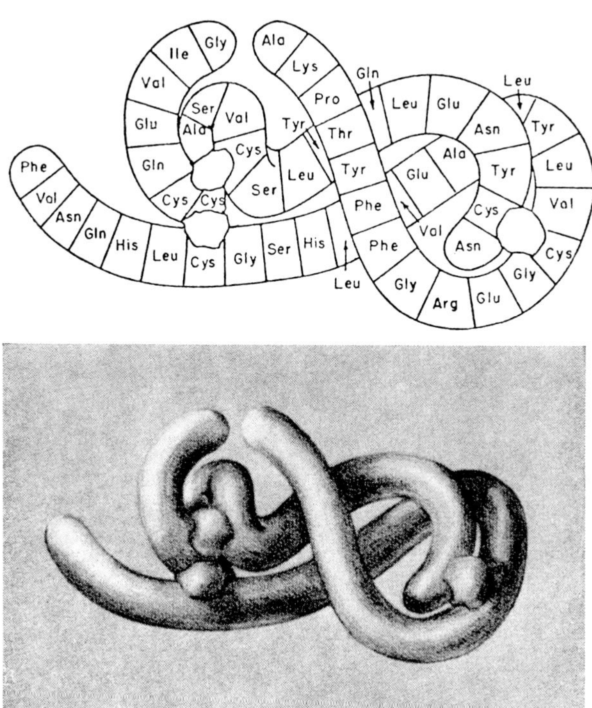

Fig. 1 b. Working models of bovine insulin (space-filling models). (From ARQUILLA, BROMER and MERCOLA, 1969)

While earlier work suggested that antigenicity was connected with high molecular weight, more recent investigations have indicated that the size of the polypeptide molecule is by no means the determining factor for its antigenicity. Polypeptides, which have a low molecular weight similar to that of insulin, show definite antigenic properties (ARNON and SELA, 1960; SELA and ARNON, 1960 a, 1960 b; SELA, 1966). Polypeptides with a large number of cyclic amino acids should therefore be prominent. This may be the reason why insulin is a stronger antigen than was previously assumed.

Other reasons for formation of antibody against insulin should be mentioned: thus, according to the view of BRUNFELDT (1966), the minutest quantity of impurities in insulin preparation is significant. Since it is recognized that proteins which are less readily soluble possess stronger immunologic properties than more soluble proteins, suspicion even fell upon the acidity of injectable insulin (DECKERT, 1966, 1968), the hormone being thought to precipitate at the injection site. By the same reasoning, the greater immunogenicity of bovine insulin as against porcine was explained by the fact that the latter can be more easily maintained in solution (SCHLICHTKRULL, 1953). Finally BERSON and YALOW (1966) have shown that insulin dissolved in weakly acid solution becomes altered (deamidition) during prolonged storage, even in the cold; thus the antigenicity is increased. In general, the technique of subcutaneous injection predetermines antibody formation. Which of these various factors is mainly responsible for the antigenicity of insulin is by no means certain.

In general, it may be said that the molecular localization of the most important immunologic (and biologic) components of the insulin molecule is no longer merely a distant prospect. Both the A and B chains possess antigenic determinants. Further details are to be found in PFEIFFER, DITSCHUNEIT and FEDERLIN (1969) (for newer concepts, see paragraph B. V).

II. Humoral Antibodies Against Insulin and Their Demonstration

From purely clinical observation the humoral insulin antibodies may be roughly divided into two groups: those which evoke allergic manifestations, and those which neutralize insulin, thereby evoking insulin resistance in certain circumstances. Considering the insulin antibodies from the point of view of demonstrability, the spectrum is expanding, as shown in Table 1.

1. Immunological Reactions and Serologic Methods

There is on the one hand the clinical observation of so-called allergic reactions of insulin antibodies in the tissue, and on the other the in-vitro method of standard serology. A severe allergic reaction,

Table 1. *Methods used for demonstration of insulin antibodies in humans and experimental animals.* (Modified from PFEIFFER, DITSCHUNEIT and FEDERLIN, 1969)

	Authors [a]
I. Hypersensitivity Reactions	
Arthus reaction	TUFT (1928)
Prausnitz-Kuestner reaction	
Schultz-Dale reaction	LEWIS (1937)
Passive cutaneous anaphylaxis	OAKLEY et al. (1959)
	DITSCHUNEIT et al. (1962)
Allergic serum transfer test	FEDERLIN and GIGLI (1968)
II. "Classical" Serological Reactions	
Precipitation	LOWELL (1942)
	LERMAN (1944)
	JONES and CUNLIFFE (1961)
Complement fixation	WASSERMAN et al. (1940)
	PAV et al. (1963)
Hemagglutination	ARQUILLA and STAVITSKY (1956)
	STEIGERWALD and SPIELMANN (1961)
	MOINAT (1958)
III. Neutralization of Biological Insulin-Effect	
"in vivo"	BANTING, FRANKS and GAIRNS (1938)
	MOLONEY and COVAL (1955)
	COLWELL and WEIGER (1956)
	ROBINSON and WRIGHT (1961)
"in vitro" on diaphragm	MARSH and HAUGAARD (1952)
	WRIGHT (1959)
"in vitro" on fat pad	RAMSEIER et al. (1961)
	SLATER et al. (1961)
	FROESCH et al. (1963)
IV. Binding of ^{131}I-Insulin to Immunoglobulins	
Separation by chromato-electrophoresis	BERSON et al. (1956)
	WELSH et al. (1956)
	MORSE (1959)
Separation by double antibody precipitation	SKOM and TALMAGE (1958)
Separation by cellulose adsorption	KERP et al. (1966)
Separation by ultra-centrifugation	KERP et al. (1970)

[a] First-named authors in teams.

evidence of the existence of IgG- or IgM-type insulin antibodies, can occur in the form of an Arthus Phenomenon, as first described by TUFT (1928). Reagins (skin-sensitizing antibodies) against insulin are demonstrated by means of the Prausnitz-Küstner technique (details in paragraph B.IV.1 concerning insulin allergy).

Utilizing the Schultz-Dale technique, LEWIS (1937) demonstrated insulin antibodies fixed in guinea-pig uterus. In the same species, WASSERMANN and MIRSKY (1942) demonstrated the existence of tissue-bound antibodies by the anaphylactic shock reaction. The susceptibility of the guinea pig to anaphylactic shock was utilized in other ways as well. OVARY 1958, 1959; OAKLEY et al. (1959) attempted to demonstrate human antibodies by means of passive cutaneous anaphylaxis; this technique was also used by DITSCHUNEIT et al. (1962). Of these reactions, virtually only the Prausnitz-Küstner technique is currently in use. Another possibility is offered by the AST-test of LAYTON, PANZANI, GREENE and CORSE (1965). Up to the present, no other method exists for the proof of reagins. Recently the demonstration of IgE antibodies in human sera by radioimmunodiffusion have been reported.

The utilization of serological methods was a further step towards the exact determination of the insulin antibodies. RICHARDSON (1938) initiated the investigation of complement-binding reactions in the serum of diabetics and normals in which he, as well as BAUER, KUNEWÄLDER and SCHÄCHTER (1937), found unspecific positive reactions in all groups. WASSERMANN, BROH-KAHN and MIRSKY (1940) were able to demonstrate in rabbits specific complement-binding antibodies against bovine insulin, these antibodies being regarded as specific. Even a retrospective study of earlier research by RAUSCH-STROOMANN and SAUER (1953), STEIGERWALD and SPIELMANN (1956) and MICHEL (1961) indicated that generally only in the rarest cases are complement-binding qualities to be found in insulin antibodies. The communications of PAV, JEZKOVA and SKRHA (1963) concerning the presence of complement-binding insulin antibodies and of PENCHEW, ANDREEW and DITZOV (1968) concerning precipitating antibodies in the serum of untreated diabetics contradict the experience of many other authors who never found such antibodies in insulin-treated diabetics. In general, the results of PAV, JEZKOVA and SKRHA (1963), of VAN DE WIEL and VAN DE WIEL-DORFMEYER (1964) with 100 normals and untreated diabetics have not been confirmed.

Even precipitation reactions, despite extensive research (review — see DECKERT, 1964) with insulin-treated diabetics, generally give negative results. Only in certain animal species have the attempts been successful: in horses (MOLONEY and APRILE, 1959) after injection of bovine insulin with Freund's adjuvant, and in guinea pigs immunized in a similar manner (JONES and CUNLIFFE, 1961; also BIRKENSHAW, RANDALL and RISDALL, 1962). HIRATA and BLUMENTHAL (1962) were able to demonstrate precipitating antibodies in guinea pigs, and occasionally in rabbits as well. ZIEGLER and LIPPMANN (1969) were successful in using goats. The passive hemagglutination technique formulated by BOYDEN (1951) is one of the most sensitive methods for detecting humoral antibodies. Thus one can successfully determine antibody-nitrogen entities at a minimum value approaching 0.005 μg (BORDUAS and GRABAR, 1953). Instead of the tannic acid technique originally used for coupling insulin onto the erythrocyte, STAVITSKY and ARQUILLA (1953) utilized bisdiazobenzidin. By this method they were able to demonstrate specifically bovine insulin antibodies in rabbits (ARQUILLA and STAVITSKY, 1956 b) and even in insulin-treated diabetics (ARQUILLA and STAVITSKY, 1956 a). Despite extensive investigations of the passive hemagglutination technique, several other authors were unable to confirm the suitability of this technique for detecting insulin antibodies in man (STEIGERWALD and SPIELMANN, 1956; STEIGERWALD et al., 1960 and especially LAPRESLE and GRABAR, 1957; further MOINAT, 1958; SCHEIFFARTH, FRENGER and MÖCKEL, 1959; MICHEL, 1961; ENGLESSON and NIELSSON, 1962). Only occasionally in some animal species, especially guinea pigs, were they able to obtain good results.

Generally speaking, one may say that these methods of classical serology are not suitable for the detection of human insulin antibodies, having been applied with success in only a few animal species, particularly guinea pigs.

2. Neutralization of the Biological Effect of Insulin

From the first investigations of DEPISCH and HASENÖRL (1928) up to the present biologic "in vivo" methods of determining insulin-neutralizing factors have been applied. The investigators mixed a certain amount of insulin with the serum of normal persons, or of diabetics, and studied the fall in blood sugar in rabbits after intravenous injection of this mixture. Lowered hypoglycemia indicated the presence of insulin-neutralizing factors.

The mouse convulsion test (BANTING, FRANK and GAIRNS, 1938) found wide application. This involves the determination of the serum amount necessary to prevent an insulin-evoked convulsion in mice. The methods were later refined by LOWELL (1944 a, b).

More exact values were obtainable by measuring the blood-sugar curve after injection of a mixture of insulin and serum (LOWELL, 1947). Variations of these methods have found application in later years (MOLONEY and COVAL, 1955; COLWELL and WEIGER, 1956; ROBINSON and WRIGHT, 1961).

A related application of measuring antibodies has been the development of methods of determining "insulin-like activity" (ILA) by the glucose consumption of the rat diaphragm, and also by the incorporation of the ^{14}C of ^{14}C-glucose into $^{14}CO_2$ in the epididymal fat pad. The serum to be investigated and a known quantity of insulin are tested on fat or muscle tissue, and the inhibition of the expected insulin-effect is calculated (SPOONT and DYER, 1951; MARSH and HAUGAARD, 1952; WRIGHT, 1959; RAMSEIER et al., 1961; SLATER et al., 1961; FROESCH et al., 1963). The methods were indeed sensitive, although inexact and unspecific for measuring antibodies.

One definitely may not equate the binding of insulin by antibodies with the neutralization of the insulin effect. The failure of correlation was discussed in detail by PFEIFFER (1966). This was very clearly shown in the experiments with the so-called Houssay dogs (SCHÖFFLING, 1966). After extirpation of the hypophysis and pancreas, an essential diminution indeed occurred, but insulin activity did not disappear from the circulatory blood (measured in fat tissue and diaphragm of the rat). Only the insulin measurable by immunologic methods disappeared from the serum directly after pancreatectomy. The so-called ILA (insulin-like activity) was still present 100 days after the operation. This could be suppressed by insulin-anti-serum both in fat tissue and in muscle.

Since, up to now, neither the molecular structure which permits the biologic effect, nor that which presents the antigenic determinants is exactly known, it is unlikely that the hormone can still be biologically active even though bound by antibody. Among the patients investigated by DITSCHUNEIT and FEDERLIN (1966), there were, for example, three cases with decreased insulin requirements but with high serum insulin-binding capacity. The metabolic balance was maintained. One can thus assume that the insulin was only weakly bound by circulating antibody. This possibility indeed was demonstrated by KERP et al. (1968) (see: Insulin resistance, B.IV.2).

3. Binding of ^{131}Iodine-labelled Insulin

A new chapter in the investigation of antibodies against insulin was initiated through the research of BERSON et al. (1956). They were able to demonstrate that ^{131}I-labelled insulin was bound by globulins in the serum of insulin-treated diabetics. By paper electrophoresis they indicated that free ^{131}I-insulin of the blood remained at the starting-point while the labelled hormone bound to the antibodies migrated with the rapid fraction of gamma globulin. These observations, which the above-mentioned authors made on patients with insulin resistance whose antibodies they wished to study, later became the beginning of the immunologic determination of insulin in the blood.

The problem of the separation of antibody-bound and free ^{131}I-insulin was solved in the following years by various investigators in different ways. While some workers made use of the differential electrophoretic mobility of the two insulin entities (BERSON et al., 1956; YALOW and BERSON, 1959; WELSH et al., 1956; MORSE, 1959), SKOM and TALMAGE (1958 a, b) precipitated the insulin-globulin complex with an antibody directed against the globulin. GRODSKY and FORSHAM (1960) achieved separation by precipitating the antibody with ammonium sulfate. MORGAN and LAZAROW (1962) precipitated the insulin in human plasma with a guinea-pig antibody. This antigen-antibody complex was again precipitated by a rabbit antibody directed against guinea-pig globulin (the double-antibody method). Similar experience was had by GOETZ et al. (1963) and HALES and RANDLE (1962).

A new approach was made by MEADE and KLITGAARD (1962) as they undertook the separation of free and bound ^{131}I-insulin by means of an ion-exchange column (Amberlite). Similar methods were also employed in the work of MELANI et al. (1965).

As determined by BERSON et al. (1956), the antigenic character of insulin is altered minimally by the weak ^{131}iodination. Since the intact insulin molecule does not enter into unspecific binding with normal serum protein, the binding of radioactively labelled insulin on the given globulins can be accepted as quite specific evidence for antibodies. Consequently, further statements may be made concerning the energy of the reactions, antibody valence, the kinetics of the antigen-antibody reaction and the molar antibody concentration. The calculation of these quantities is based upon the concept of the antigen-antibody action as a reversible bimolecular reaction, and its obedience to the Law of Mass Effect (ARRHENIUS and MADSEN, 1903). Thus, between the concentration of the antigen-antibody complex and the product of the concentration of free antibody and free antigen, there is always a definite proportion of equivalent weight which is dependent upon the reaction constant. These proportions of equivalent weight can be measured experimentally and yield information concerning the energy liberated by the reaction of antigen with antibody, and therefore also the strength of binding.

Utilizing definite small antigens and applying the Law of Mass Effect, it has been shown that an antibody molecule always contains two valences which, however, react with the antigen with varying degrees of intensity (EISEN and KARUSH, 1949; CARSTEN and EISEN, 1955; NISONOFF and PRESSMAN, 1958). Every antibody is therefore heterogeneous.

Occasionally so-called "natural" antibodies appear to be homogeneous with regard to their reaction constants, in contrast to immune antibodies. Homogenous immunoglobulins are also found in multiple myeloma, myasthenia gravis and in cold-agglutination.

The heterogeneity of the antibodies against insulin was proved experimentally by BERSON and YALOW (1959 a, b). This heterogeneity is expressed in the fact that the proportion of bound to free ^{131}I insulin ($^{B}/_{F}$) relative to antibody-bound unlabelled insulin (B) is subject to an exponential regularity, and hence describes a rising concave curve. These reaction curves enabled the maximum insulin-binding capacity of the serum to be determined for both antibody-binding sites, and their respective proportionality contents could be calculated from the experimental data. The concept of these reaction curves further permitted the quantitative determination of cross-reactions of an insulin antibody with insulins of different species.

(For further details see DECKERT, 1964; PFEIFFER, DITSCHUNEIT and FEDERLIN, 1969).

4. The Types of Insulin Antibodies

The insulin-binding antibodies of the neutralizing type in human beings belong in general to immunoglobulins of the class IgG. This has been observed in diabetics by several authors (Morse and Heremans, 1962; Yagi et al., 1963; Chao, Karam and Grodsky, 1965; Toro-Goyca, Martinez-Maldonald and Matos, 1966; Devlin and O'Donovan, 1966). At the initiation of antibody formation, antibodies of the type IgM have also been demonstrated (Samols and Jones, 1965; Devlin, 1966; Kerp, 1968; Yagi et al., 1963). These could be found from the second day of insulin therapy, persisting to the 43rd day (Devlin). Yagi et al. (1963) and Cerasi et al. (1966) observed insulin binding of IgA in patients with generalized immediate allergic response (systemic hypersensitivity). Patterson, Roberts and Pruzansky (1969) have reported findings which indicate that the reaginic antibody to an insulin-allergic subject was in an immunoglobulin class other than IgG, IgA and IgM. Recently Dolovich et al. (1970) were able to demonstrate the presence of IgE antibodies to bovine insulin in a patient with generalized allergic reactions. Therefore it is very probable that insulin antibodies with reagin-activity belong to this newly discovered class of immunoglobulins (Ishizaka, Ishizaka and Hornbrook, 1966) as it has been shown for nearly all the other antibodies which are responsible for immediate reactions. Finally the detection of IgD antibodies to insulin in three of six diabetics has been reported (Devey, Carter, Sanderson and Coombs, 1970). The authors used the red-blood-cell linked antigen-antiglobulin reaction. Compared with the IgG titres the IgD antibody titres were low.

III. Cell Mediated Immunity Against Insulin

1. Some General Aspects of Cell Mediated Immunity

This form of immunological response and the cellular events which accompany it involves the formation of a population of sensitized cells. These cells are primarily lymphocytes which possess the property, apparently independent of extra-cellular antibody, of specifically interacting with the antigen so as to elicit the phenomenon of delayed-type hypersensitivity. They belong to a population of small lymphocytes which is controlled by the thymus (called T lymphocytes, i. e. thymus-dependent lymphocytes), in contrast to the thymus-independent lymphocytes (B lymphocytes, i. e. bursa-dependent lymphocytes) which later proliferate to become the antibody-producing plasma cells. Between the B and T lymphocytes there occurs an intercellular contact process which enhances antibody formation by the B lymphocytes.

T lymphocytes are able specifically to react with an antigenic determinant of the immunogen and are capable of producing a delayed immune reaction after intradermal injection of antigen. This phenomenon cannot be attributed to antibodies synthesized by other cells and subsequently transferred to these lymphocytes but rather to some built-in property of the lymphocytes themselves. There is much evidence that certain cells among the antigen-sensitive lymphocytes bear immunoglobulins on their surface (Reviewed by ROITT et al., 1969). These cells, termed "actively allergized" cells by COOMBS and LACHMANN (1968), must be distinguished from those which absorb antibodies passively, as in the case of cytophilic antibodies (see also, C.I.6.δ).

Cell mediated specific immunity occurs typically when the immunogenic stimulus is a living allograft or when a small quantity of an inert immunogen is deposited in a depot (e. g. in the skin) from which it is only slowly released. Some of the properties of sensitized lymphocytes can be used to demonstrate the state of cell mediated immunity.

a) Specific contact between antigen and sensitized lymphocytes has frequently been observed. It has been demonstrated in various models employing different techniques. ROSENAU and MOON (1961) and KOPROWSKI and FERNANDES (1962) showed the reaction of lymphocytes from sensitized animals with target cells from tissue culture. Using an indirect method, GILLISSEN (1963, 1964) demonstrated complement binding of antigen reactive cells in tuberculin sensitized animals. A further step is the ability to demonstrate rosette formation in vitro with small lymphocytes after sensitization to sheep erythrocytes (NOTA, LIACOPOULOS-BRIOT, STIFFEL and BIOZZI, 1964); even for insulin (FREI, CRUCHAUD and VANOTTI, 1965) showed such a rosette phenomenon of delayed hypersensitivity to insulin with insulin coated erythrocytes and sensitized blood lymphocytes. Of special interest for the present work are investigations measuring the uptake of labelled antigen by lymphocytes. WITTEN, WANG and KILLIAN (1963) were able to demonstrate that a significantly greater number of the circulating lymphocytes were stained by fluorescein-conjugated PPD (purified protein derivative) in patients with a positive skin test to PPD (about 4% of lymphocytes) than in patients with a negative reaction (about 0.5%). HJORT, BEUTNER and WITEBSKY (1968) showed that delayed hypersensitivity of rabbits to PPD was accompanied by the capacity of peripheral blood lymphocytes to react with fluorescein-labelled PPD (controls: 0—1%; sensitized animals after skin test: 3—7%). To summarize, one can assume that, in the condition of delayed hypersensitivity, the sensitized white blood cells contain surface receptors which enable them to recognize their specific antigen. Against this background, a demonstration will be sought that insulin-sensitized cells exist in the blood of patients with delayed allergic skin reactions to insulin.

b) Another in vitro reaction of sensitized lymphocytes was observed in their ability to differentiate and divide under the influence of antigen, a reaction similar to that evoked by mitogenic agents like PHA (phytohemagglutinin) but less marked and involving a smaller proportion of lymphocytes. However, at the present, it is not quite clear whether this transformation is correlated only with the presence of cell mediated immunity or also with circulating antibody.

c) Interaction between sensitized lymphocytes and specific antigen can be demonstrated with the migration inhibition test. The migration of macrophages of either the sensitized or the unsensitized animal is inhibited by a factor released from the sensitized lymphocytes in the presence of antigen (see paragraph D.I.1.d).

d) Finally, cellular immunity can be transferred to another organism by means of living lymphocytes, or in the case of tuberculosis, by their extract — the so-called transfer factor (LAWRENCE, 1949, 1955, 1960), as the essential cell substance.

The morphological picture of delayed hypersensitivity shows a chronic inflammation which could be caused by a number of different pathological processes. The cellular infiltrate of these reactions is not specific to the hypersensitivity but is determined by the manner in which particular tissues of a certain species react to any irritant process of the same intensity and over the same period of time (TURK, 1967). The histological pattern depends on the species — there are marked differences — and on the antigen. Nevertheless the tissue changes show many similarities. Some details are mentioned later in chapter E.III. in connection with autoimmune conditions.

Relationship to Antibody Production. At present, delayed hypersensitivity is regarded as an immunologic mechanism which is independent of antibody production, in spite of the close relationship between the two immune responses. It could be shown that they can coexist although the delayed immune reaction can be masked when appreciable amounts of antibody are being produced. Nevertheless according to COOMBS and GELL (1968) "it would appear that delayed allergy is related, in some way which is still obscure, to the inductive and proliferative phases of the immunological processes, while antibody production is of course related to the productive, or rather to the mass-productive phases."

Nomenclature. Finally it is necessary to mention and define the nomenclature used in the present work in connection with the immune reaction of the delayed type. The terms "delayed allergy" or "delayed allergic reaction" are used to describe a skin reaction which appears with a delay of 18—24 hours (in contrast to the immediate reaction which occurs within 15—30 minutes after the application of an antigen). The terms "delayed immune reaction", "cellular immunity", "cell-mediated immune response", "delayed hypersensitivity" are used as synonyms for the immune reaction itself which is due to the presence of sensitized lymphocytes (type IV reaction as described by COOMBS and GELL, 1968). According to HUMPHREY and WHITE (1970) cell-mediated immunity "is used to describe the appearance of a heightened reactivity towards the antigen manifested by such phenomena as delayed type hypersensitivity and rejection of foreign tissue grafts." Nevertheless it should be mentioned that the use of the terms "allergic" or "allergy" in this respect would be more accurate than the terms "immune" or "immunity" which suggest protection, as described in detail by COOMBS and GELL.

2. Previous Immunocytological Studies

The number of investigations concerning humoral antibodies against insulin, in man as well as in animals, is in marked contrast to the few reports of the detection of insulin antibodies in or on cells. Intracellular antibodies against insulin were found by PARKER, ELEVITCH and GRODSKY (1963) in guinea pigs immunized to bovine or porcine insulin, together with Freund's adjuvant. By means of insulin marked with fluorescein-isothiocyanate, the authors demonstrated the binding of the antigen on plasma cells in lymph nodes and spleen. Thus the proof was obtained for "humoral antibodies" which were still detectable in the cell, as described with various other antigens, by means of immunofluorescence (COONS, LEDUC and CONOLLY, 1955; LEDUC, COONS and CONOLLY, 1955; WHITE, COONS and CONOLLY, 1955; WHITE, 1954; VASQUEZ, 1961).

In humans, the immunologically specific binding of insulin by cells was first observed by KERP, STEINHILBER, KIELING and CREUTZFELDT (1965). The proof was carried out, not directly on the cell, but on the cellular extract from a mixture of circulating leukocytes. In one case of delayed local sensitivity to insulin, the authors were able to determine a clearly increased binding capacity of insulin. Shortly after this, FREI, CRUCHAUD and VANNOTTI (1965) observed a case of delayed local insulin sensitivity, in whose serum no humoral antibodies were found. The skin test indicated a delayed immunological reaction, and isolated leukocytes from the patient's blood reacted, in a small amount (15.5 per 1000), by the formation of rosettes after the addition of insulin-fixed erythrocytes. No special investigations were undertaken of the type of leukocytes involved.

IV. Clinical Symptoms of the Immune Response to Insulin

1. Insulin Allergy

Even in the first year of insulin therapy, allergic reactions to insulin were observed. Four of the eighty-three diabetics first treated with insulin developed urticarial skin lesions (JOSLIN, GRAY and ROOT, 1922). Although at that time it was a question of preparation, the insulin being very likely contaminated with numerous other animal proteins which were long held accountable for the allergic symptoms, some such side-effects are still observed with the highly purified insulin now in use. Hence, they do not arise as a simple consequence of impurities (but see paragraph B. V).

a) The Clinical Picture

Allergic symptoms after parenteral administration of insulin are mostly observed in the skin. The organism can, however, react in rare

Table 2. *Classification of insulin allergy by* PALEY *and* TUNBRIDGE. (From MARBLE, 1959)

1. Mild Local Reactions.
   A. Immediate
      (1) Stinging on injection (by no means an invariable occurrence).
      (2) Swelling and redness appear 1—2 hours after injection.
      (3) Area of reaction 1—4 cm. in diameter.
      (4) Maximum intensity 12—24 hours after injection.
      (5) Disappears in 1—3 days.
   B. Delayed
      Similar to the immediate reaction, but onset delayed 6 to 24 hours after injection.

2. Severe Local Reactions.
   A. Immediate
      (1) Observed within 1 hour of injection.
      (2) Area involved may extend to 15 cm. in diameter.
      (3) Usually disappears within a week.
   B. Delayed
      Identical with previous reaction, but onset delayed 6 to 24 hours after injection.

3. Generalized Reactions.
   Not encountered in series of PALEY and TUNBRIDGE.

4. Pseudo-Reactions.

cases with other "target organs". The most frequent symptoms are local in nature. At the injection site occur burning, itching, painful sensations, together with reddening, swelling, and heat, rarely immediate, mostly after a few hours, or even days. The affected area varies in size, generally from 1 to 4 cm., although even larger areas have been observed. The reaction reaches its height in 24—36 hours and recedes after 2—3 days. But the symptoms vary widely in regard to time of initial outset and intensity and duration. They are classified by MARBLE (1959 a) according to a scheme based on the clinical aspects by PALEY and TUNBRIDGE (1952): Table 2.

While the local reactions generally recede without sequelae, in very rare cases skin necrosis can follow, i. e. an Arthus phenomenon as described by TUFT (1928), BARTELHEIMER (1952), SCHIRREN (1953),

Porter and Hartmann (1970). The patient observed by Kulpe (1958) developed sensitivity to Surfen. In some patients prolonged insulin therapy evokes certain skin changes, described by Adam (1960) as follows: "... firm, for the most part painful, red or blue-red knots of lentil or cherry-size, which affect the cutis and occasionally the dermis, which exist for periods of weeks or months and can heal leaving atrophic scars. Under these circumstances these regions, which were preferentially utilized for injection, present a colorful picture: young and old, i. e. larger and smaller, tumors in a color saturation between red and blue, interspersed with atrophic cutaneous areas and localized pigmentation. There can also be firm, nodular infiltrates with a hard epidermal covering, which not only is cosmetically disturbing but also means varying resorption ability for insulin ..." Whether these lesions — so frequently seen in every diabetic center — have an allergic basis, is still open to question. Scheffler (1955) was able to demonstrate iron-containing pigment and malanin in the peculiar brown-red pigmented cutaneous areas of one patient. Perhaps there is an equal uncertainty about the allergic origin of insulin lipodystrophy (complete review by Boulin-Chimenes and Tourneur, 1952; Kehrer, 1949; and Marble, 1959 b).

In comparison with the above-mentioned local lesions, generalized insulin reactions are far less frequent. The generalized reaction complex involves urticaria, pruritus, Quincke edema, joint swelling, fever, exanthema, stomach and intestinal lesions, asthma and also serious anaphylactic shock.

While Marble (1959) at the Joslin Clinic in Boston observed no fatal cases, Hansen (1957) and Miller (1962) reported several fatalities. A unique case is the observation of a serious thrombocytopenic purpura by Constam (1956), also the observation of Boulin et al. (1955) of a disseminated panarteritis. Very recently the combination of insulin resistance and thrombocytopenic purpura in the same patient was observed (Cawley and Browne, 1970).

b) Frequency

Reports of the frequency of allergic cutaneous symptoms reflect a great variability. Thus, Allan and Scherer (1932) reported from a study of 18,000 diabetics that 14% of patients reacted allergically. In contrast, Paley and Tunbridge (1952) gave the figure of 55.8%.

These authors did not have the population study of the former; indeed, they surveyed only 147 patients. Women are more frequently affected than men. These reports indicated further that the majority of reactions are of a mild nature (80—85%) and predominantly immediate.

Marble (1959 a), from his experience with patients at the Joslin Clinic, stated that perhaps 25—33% of insulin-treated patients observe an allergic reaction once at some time in their treatment. This figure stands between those of Allan and Scherer, and Paley and Tunbridge.

Certainly puzzling are the observations of Arkins, Engbring and Lennon (1962) concerning subcutaneous testing and an associated tendency to allergic reaction. Arkins et al. found a positive skin reaction in 40 out of a total of 76 patients. Surprisingly, 3 out of 29 patients who had never received insulin reacted positively.

The number of reports of generalized reactions is remarkably small. Andreani and Corti (1955) wrote of 3 cases among 1522 insulin-tested diabetics, i. e. 0.2%. Hansen (1957) estimated that generalized reactions constituted 1% of all the allergic reactions associated with insulin. In some instances these can occur very soon after therapy is started. Rose and Barron (1955) reported a case of anaphylactic shock after 11 days, and Walker (1926) reported a similar case that had occurred only 3 days after the initial injection. More serious generalized reactions occur relatively often among nondiabetics, according to the work of Dahl (1950). Indeed, he observed 7 instances of anaphylactic reaction in 1108 psychiatric patients receiving shock therapy (0.6%), and without exception these were women at the time of the menses.

Paley and Tunbridge (1952) had reported earlier on the frequency of allergic reactions in women after insulin therapy: 65% of the women patients and only 26% of the men developed allergic skin reactions.

c) Etiology and Pathogenesis

A few years ago it was assumed that these allergic manifestations could be derived from 1. insulin itself; 2. foreign protein of the animal source; 3. impurities; 4. additives, especially of a protein nature, such as protamine or globin (Marble, 1959 a). Primarily the impurities were impugned, and probably justly so in those early years of insulin therapy (Hansen and Eyer, 1933). However, the opinion persisted that *only* the impurities, and not insulin itself, were the cause of allergic reactions (Jorpes, 1949). He had shown in quite thorough studies of 300 diabetics with insulin allergy, that the skin symptoms disappeared after the introduction of (multiple) recrystallized insulin. Hagen and Hagen (1959) expressed a similar opinion. They tested the intracutaneous reaction of various insulin preparations, having proved this method of application as a test for tissue compatibility in previous investigations (Hagen et al., 1958). It appeared that the degree of purification of the insulin preparations was largely responsible for this intracutaneous compatibility, which, however, proved not to be dependent upon the number of recrystallizations. Simple recrystallized insulin ("Novo") was indeed almost as compatible as triple recrystallized insulin. On the other hand, there was no doubt that the antigenic effect of an injected insulin dose was less, the greater the degree of purification. The recent detection of proinsulin and other components in the extract of the β-cells throws new light upon the theory of "impurities" in insulin (see B. V).

Humoral insulin antibodies are thought to be responsible for the acute allergic phenomena of local or generalized type. Loveless and Cann (1953) could not effect an exact classification of reagins to definite groups of immunoglobulins. Lachnit and Wiedemann (1961) demonstrated thermolabile reagins, which were not 7S globulins, in a severe local immediate allergy. These reagins could be demonstrated by the antiglobulin consumption test.

Heremans and Vaerman (1962) found a specific activity in the region of the IgA globulins in a patient with generalized immediate allergy. Yagi et al. (1963) demonstrated a skin-sensitizing activity, not only by IgA but also by IgM globulins, while other authors held the IgG and IgA globulins responsible for allergic symptoms (Rivera, Toro-Goyko and Matos, 1965). In the more recent investigations of Devlin and O'Donovan (1965) also of Devlin (1966, 1968), the isolated appearance of IgM globulins in patients with localized immediate allergy against insulin is reported. The newly discovered IgE-antibodies against insulin in a case of generalized allergy has already been mentioned (see B.II.4). These investigations are concerned exclusively with the acute forms of insulin allergy. The clinically more frequent delayed local reactions have barely been investigated so far.

2. Insulin Resistance

Besides the several forms of insulin allergy, another consequence of the production of antibodies against insulin is insulin resistance. This topic is not central to this monograph but, being part of the main theme, "immunopathology of insulin", should be briefly explained. (Factors leading to so-called "tissue resistance" to insulin and which act as inhibitors of insulin activity, like free fatty acids, certain fractions of plasma proteins and hormonal antagonists including adrenal corticosteroids, STH, ACTH, placental lactogen, glucagon, catecholamines and thyroxine will not be considered here.)

Martin, Martin, Lyster and Strouse (1941) defined insulin resistance as an insulin requirement exceeding 200 U/24 hr over at least a 48-hr period. The amount of insulin required by primarily nondiabetic but later pancreatectomized patients is between 26 and 42 U/24 hr (Waugh et al., 1946; Creutzfeldt, Kern, Kümmerle and Schumacher, 1961). Therefore any higher requirement of insulin to maintain normal blood sugar levels to some extent indicates insulin resistance. It thus appears more logical that a requirement of 100 U/24 hr can also be accepted as resistance, which embraces a considerably larger group of patients.

a) Clinical Picture

The increase in insulin requirement takes place gradually without obvious causes over a period of weeks or months, seldom within a shorter time. Resistance occurs in adults but also in children (Guthrie and Womack, 1967). The daily insulin requirement can reach extremely high values. Pfeiffer (1966) described a daily dose of 40,000 U. Tucker et al. (1964) even a maximum of 177,580 U. It is not possible to predict the course of the resistance. Despite high doses of insulin, the glucose metabolism may be under control. On the other hand, the insulin requirement can spontaneously fall to very low levels, causing severe hypoglycemia (Oberdisse, 1948; Morse, 1961).

b) Frequency

True resistance according to the criteria of Martin et al. (1941) may be expected in about 0.1% of all insulin-treated diabetics (Shipp, Cunningham, Russel and Marble, 1965; Daweke, 1966; Devlin,

1968). However, the incidence seems to vary greatly between different countries and nations. In Denmark insulin resistance is rare (Schlichtkrull, 1967); Deckert observed not a single case of insulin resistance among 3000 diabetics. In our own population of diabetics, 40 out of 1089 (i. e. 3.6%) needed more than 100 U/day (Ditschuneit and Federlin, 1966). The reasons for these great differences are still unknown but are being studied.

c) *Methods for Measurement of Insulin-neutralizing Antibodies*

Insulin antibodies of the neutralizing type can be measured by various techniques. The mouse convulsion test shows in vivo the neutralizing effect of a patient's serum on the shock-evoking action of a definite amount of insulin (Banting, Frank and Gairns, 1938; Moloney and Goldsmith, 1957). The neutralization of the insulin activity by antibodies can also be measured in vitro through glucose uptake — or oxidation of the isolated diaphragm or epididymal fat pad of the rat (Pfeiffer and Ditschuneit, 1962). Another technique makes use of the binding of the antigen in vivo by the patient's serum. The decrease of radioactivity in the blood is tested after injection of 1 U ^{131}iodine-labelled insulin intravenously (Williams et al., 1953; Welsh, Henly, Williams and Cox, 1956; Berson et al., 1956; Pfeiffer and Ditschuneit, 1962). The classical serological methods cannot be used for the determination of insulin antibodies in humans. In contrast to their practicability in some species of animals, in humans they have seldom been employed with real success (Lowell, 1942; 1944; Lerman, 1944; Moinat, 1958; Loveless and Cann, 1955; Arquilla and Stavitsky, 1956 b).

Not until the use of ^{131}iodine-labelled insulin (Kallee, 1952) by Berson et al. (1956) for the demonstration of insulin binding of serum in vitro was it possible to measure quantitatively the amount of antibodies and their maximum binding capacity. The authors showed that the binding of insulin to its antibody is a reversible process and that, with constant antibody concentration, the ratio of bound to free insulin was an inverse function of the insulin concentration. In further work by Berson and Yalow (1959 a, b) the quantitative relationships in the reaction between insulin and its antibodies was extensively researched. It was shown that insulin antibodies have stronger and weaker binding areas for the antigen. This made it possible to measure the maximum binding capacity of a patient's serum for insulin. With special binding curves (see Fig. 2) the binding can be determined for insulin of different species, including human insulin. BERSON and YALOW (1959 a) recognized in the serum of non-resistant insulin-treated patients binding capacities of not more than 10 U/liter, whereas in patients with resistance the amount was 50 and sometimes in excess of 500 U/liter.

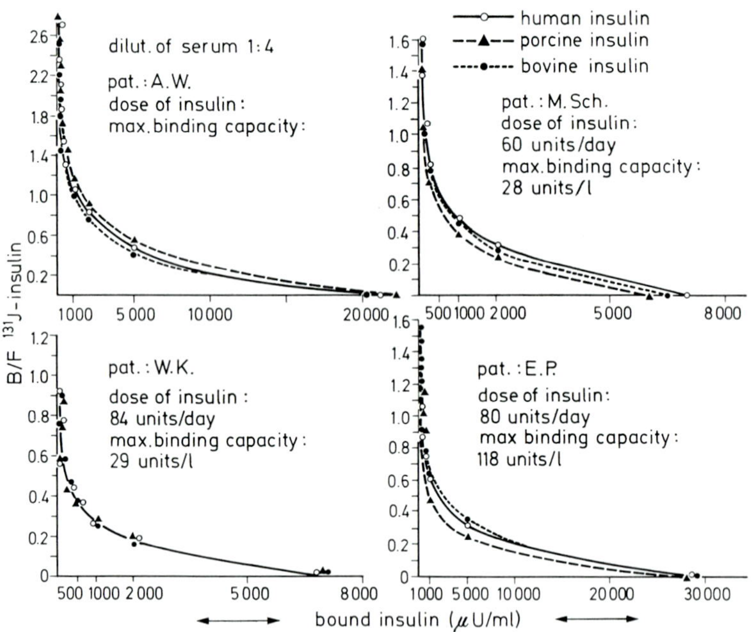

Fig. 2. Quotient of bound to free ¹³¹iodine labelled bovine insulin in relation to the amounts of bound insulin from different species. (From DITSCHUNEIT and FEDERLIN, 1966)

The binding of human sera for bovine and ovine insulin was stronger than for porcine or equine insulin (BERSON and YALOW, 1959 b). Human insulin showed weaker cross reactions than insulin of the animal species. Apart from the fact that some authors expressed a few objections from the technical point of view (KERP et al., 1966; BRUNFELDT, 1966; DEVLIN, 1968), the method of BERSON and YALOW has so far proved to be a most useful technique.

d) Relationships between Maximum Insulin-binding Capacity of the Serum and the Daily Requirement of Insulin

A correlation between insulin requirement and insulin-binding capacity in serum is found in many, though not all, insulin-treated diabetics (BERSON and YALOW, 1959 a; ROSSELIN et al., 1965; DITSCHUNEIT and FEDERLIN, 1966). In contrast, the association constants of strong and weak binding areas of insulin antibodies exhibit no recognizable correlation with insulin requirement (DITSCHUNEIT and FEDERLIN, 1966; KERP, KASEMIR and KIELING, 1968). KERP et al. found a significant dependence of the daily insulin requirement upon the concentration of the stronger binding component AK_1 (antibody component 1) and a lower dependence upon the weaker binding component AK_2 (antibody component 2). Furthermore, it was shown by these authors that patients with a low insulin requirement but relatively high maximum insulin-binding capacity of the serum had a higher concentration of AK_2 than of AK_1. Obviously insulin which is bound to antibody-binding components of this type retains its biological activity. This would explain the often observed phenomenon that, in spite of high serum values of maximum insulin-binding capacity, the organism retains its insulin sensitivity.

KASEMIR, PAULUS, STEINHILBER and KERP (1968) observed in patients treated with mixed insulins (bovine-porcine) that bovine insulin was preferentially bound to the stronger binding antibody component whereas more porcine insulin was bound to the weaker binding antibody component. This observation may explain why porcine insulin is repeatedly found to be more effective in patients with insulin resistance. More detailed information about insulin resistance is given by FEDERLIN, DITSCHUNEIT and PFEIFFER (1971). (For insulin antibodies in general see DECKERT, 1964; DEVLIN, 1968; PFEIFFER, DITSCHUNEIT and FEDERLIN, 1969).

V. Proinsulin and Newer Concepts in Insulin Immunology

In the following part a series of clinical and experimental results from several years' work is presented. As far as possible the observations are linked to recognized theories and hypotheses. Scientific progress is so rapid that new developments tend to extend (or reduce) the value of results. This is also true of the immunopathology of insulin, as regards both insulin itself and the immunological reactions which we have investigated.

Therefore an assessment of the present situation is imperative before this brief review of the immunology of insulin is closed. Of primary importance is the discovery of proinsulin by STEINER (1967) and his group. Extending their studies of the biosynthesis of insulin by islet-cell tumors (STEINER and OYER, 1967; STEINER, CUNNING-

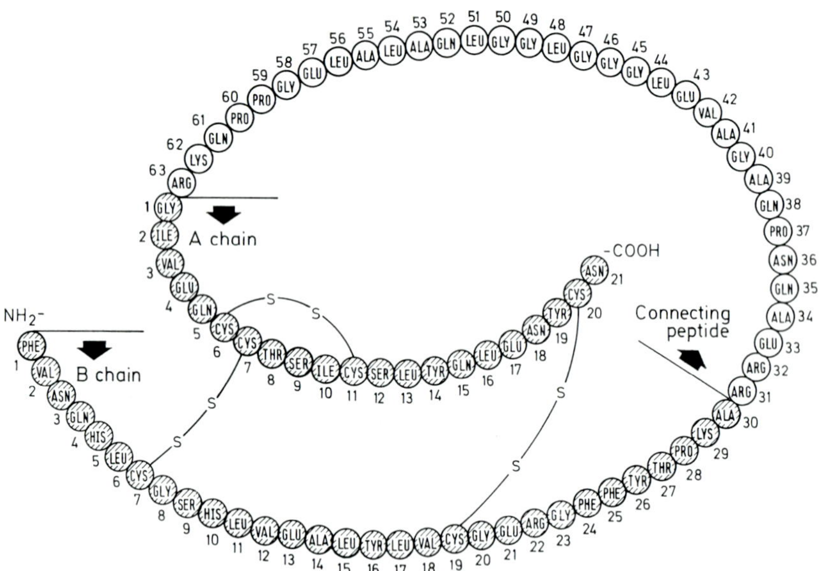

Fig. 3 a. Amino-acid sequence of porcine proinsulin. (From SHAW and CHANCE, 1968)

HAM, SPIGELMAN and ATEN, 1967), the authors demonstrated that insulin is formed from a precursor of higher molecular weight which has been named proinsulin. Proinsulin consists of a single polypeptide chain (see Fig. 3 a), beginning with the N-terminal of the B chain and continuing through the so-called "connecting peptide" to the N-terminal of the A chain. The A and B chains are already linked with each other at designated locations through disulfide bonds. The task of proinsulin in the cell appears to be to facilitate the formation of disulfide bonds (STEINER and CLARK, 1968). Later the C-peptide is split off in the cell. Whether proinsulin also has an extracellular function is not yet certain. First reports show that proinsulin appears in small amounts in the serum of diabetics (RUBENSTEIN, CHO and STEINER, 1968) and in normal and obese subjects (MELANI, RUBENSTEIN and STEINER, 1970). Also the C-peptide portion of proinsulin is secreted along with insulin and circulates in the blood. —

The biological activity of bovine proinsulin in isolated fat cells is only about 2% that of insulin (GLIEMANN, 1967; GLIEMANN and MOODY, 1968). Utilizing porcine proinsulin in rats, SHAW and CHANCE (1968) detected no biologic effect upon epididymal fat tissue and diaphragm. Recently STEINER et al. (1970) reported that proinsulin, when injected into animals, exhibits biologic activity of the order of 15—30 per cent that of insulin.

Proinsulin has been identified by several research groups in insulin preparations from cattle, pig, rat and human pancreas. It amounts to (on average) some 2% of the total protein of the preparation investigated (STEINER, HALLUND, RUBENSTEIN, CHO and BAYLISS, 1968). In addition to proinsulin, what is thought to be an intermediate form has been identified in cattle by STEINER et al. (1968); this substance is composed of proinsulin molecules which themselves represent split products from the amino-acid binding sites on the A chain. According to SCHLICHTKRULL et al. (1969) several substances are distinguishable in crystalline porcine insulin by means of polyacrylamide gel electrophoresis, among them:

1. monodesamide insulin
2. insulin and the dimer
3. intermediate
4. arginine insulin
5. proinsulin
6. an as-yet uncharacterized substance

By means of gel filtration (Sephadex G 50), these authors fractionated crystalline insulin into a-, b- and c-components. The a-component is probably of exocrine origin, while the b-component consists of proinsulin, intermediate and the dimer, and the c-component is principally insulin itself, the so-called monocomponent insulin.

A comparison of the proinsulins of various species reveals that these differ from one another in the number and sequence of amino acids to a greater extent than the pure insulin molecule. The reason for this is the different composition of the C-peptide which consists of 30 (bovine) or 33 (porcine) amino acids connecting the A and B chains (STEINER et al., 1968; CHANCE et al., 1968; SCHMIDT and ARENS, 1968). In general the two proinsulins differ even in the amino acid sequence — in 30% (RUBENSTEIN, et al., 1969). The human C-peptide sequence also differs substantially from that of the porcine or bovine molecules (OYER, CHO and STEINER, 1970) (see Fig. 3 b).

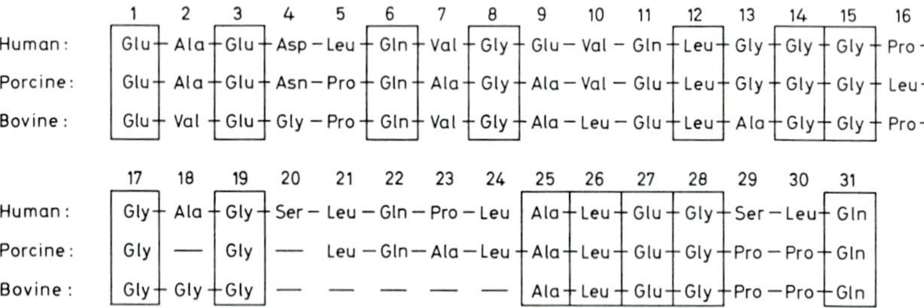

Fig. 3 b. Primary structures of human, porcine and bovine proinsulin C-peptides. The amino acids which are identical in all three C-peptides are enclosed; they comprise about 50% of the amino acids. Because of the differences in length of the C-peptides in these species arbitrary deletions are made to enable the best comparisons. (From MELANI, RUBENSTEIN, OYER and STEINER, 1970)

A reflection of these differences is given by the high degree of immunologic specificity of the reaction with proinsulin antisera. After the removal of antibodies directed against insulin these antisera do not react with insulin or proinsulin from other species. For the specific detection of human proinsulin in serum samples therefore it was necessary to develop an immuno-assay system directed against its C-peptide determinants. Because C-peptide alone did not results in antibody production in guinea pigs it was necessary to couple the antigen to a larger protein such as rabbit albumin. By this method it was possible to get antibodies that reacted strongly with human proinsulin and human C-peptide (MELANI, RUBENSTEIN, OYER and STEINER, 1970). Because of the presence of both proinsulin and C-peptide in blood and the cross reactivity of these proteins in the human C-peptide immunoassay system, direct measurement of these proteins in unextracted serum was not yet possible. The authors needed a preliminary separation of the proteins by gel filtration. Perhaps in the future direct measurement of proinsulin will be possible because it could be shown by STOLL, TOUBER, ENSINCK and WILLIAMS (1970) that guinea pigs are able to develop antibodies to porcine proinsulin which did not react significantly with either insulin or C-peptide.

The immunological characteristics of the substances isolated from crystallized insulin are of particular interest. If one assumes in accordance with the data given above that only the hormone insulin itself, C-peptide and small amounts of proinsulin are secreted by the B cell, then it follows that injection of extracted (crystalline) insulin introduces substances to which the homologous organism would be expected to have no immunologic tolerance. Thus antibody formation to "insulin" may be directed more against the insulin-related proteins than against the essential hormone. This would explain why antibody formation to bovine insulin can be stimulated in cattle (RENOLD, SOELDNER and STEINKE, 1964) (see: chapter E.), to porcine insulin in pigs (BRUNFELDT and DECKERT, 1964), to ovine insulin in sheep (RENOLD et al., 1965) and even to human insulin in humans (DECKERT and GRUNDAHL, 1969). In the heterologous system antibody formation may be enhanced by the discrepancy in the chemical structure of proinsulin. Yet immunization studies in guinea pigs showed that the immunogenicity of proinsulin compared with that of insulin was not very different (WRIGHT and MAKULU, 1969; FEDERLIN, 1970; KERP, STEINHILBER and SCHMIDT, 1970). On the other hand rabbits immunized with crystalline proinsulin from pigs in small doses (40 μg) formed antibodies which were able to bind insulin to a considerably greater extent than animals immunized with twenty times the dose of crystalline bovine insulin (SCHLICHTKRULL et al., 1969). The same authors found that pure monocomponent insulin did not evoke antibody formation in these animals. Of further interest were the observations that the a-component isolated from crystalline insulin — the presumptive exocrine component — was particularly antigenic and that even the dimer insulin evoked antibody formation.

As the conclusion from their results SCHLICHTKRULL and his coworkers stated that the neutralization of the biological effect of injected insulin from foreign species in human diabetics is due to antibodies which are directed against proinsulin and its related proteins but crossreact with the pure hormone. First investigations of the immunogenic role of proinsulin in patients treated with commercial insulin led to contradictory results. DITSCHUNEIT, HINZ and FAULHABER (1969) showed preferential binding of the antibodies in serum to proinsulin. HINKE, STEINHILBER, SCHMIDT and KERP (1970) found higher concentrations of antibody-binding sites to insulin than to proinsulin in patients treated with bovine insulin. Further studies by this group regarding the reaction between bovine insulin or bovine proinsulin and insulin-(proinsulin-)binding antibodies do not confirm the hypothesis that proinsulin in commercial insulin preparations is an essential stimulus for insulin antibody production (KERP, STEINHILBER and KASEMIR, 1970). On the other hand SCHLICHTKRULL (1970) reported that in diabetic patients no antibodies or only insignificant amounts were formed during treatment for several months with insulin preparations made from monocomponent (i. e. "pure") insulin. This seems to offer the hope that the immunological side effects of insulin therapy might be reduced by this purified insulin; whether they will be eliminated must remain open.

For further studies of the immunological properties of proinsulin and c-peptide see: KITABCHI, A. E.: J. clin. Invest. **49,** 979 (1970).

Notes added in proof (regarding the structure of insulin)

In attempting to investigate the stereochemical and thermodynamic permissibilities on numerous correctly proportioned molecular models of insulin, it was found that the guanidinium group of arginine (B. 22.) can form a strong resonating ionic linkage with asparagine (A.21.). This conformation appears to cover the interchain disulphide bridges CyS (A 20)—CyS (B.19) and therefore could afford partial protection against rupture. Rupture of this ionic bond may occur on addition of other guanidinium group-containing compounds such as protamines, or doubly positively charged cations such as Zn^2, or doubly negatively charged multioxyanions such as sulphate. The rupture of this ionic bond involves exposure of these groups, hence the antigenicity of insulin may well be altered. This, in fact, is known to occur with sulphated insulin. (LEWIN, S.: Insulin conformations. Biochem. J. **114,** 83 p, 1969).

C. Investigations of Insulin Allergy in Diabetics

I. Investigations of Delayed Insulin Allergy

1. Introductory Remarks

It will be clear from the previous chapter concerning the clinical forms of insulin allergy that allergic reactions of the immediate type, with local or generalized manifestations, are relatively rare observed.

In contrast, the delayed-onset reaction is a much more frequent but fleeting occurrence, often even sub-threshold. The pathogenesis remains unexplained. The fact that these allergic reactions occur after a few injections, i. e. at the beginning of the immunization, mostly with a latency period of 12 to 24 hours, and cease after 24—48 hours suggests the descriptive classification: "delayed-onset allergic reaction." The assumption that this represents the state of delayed hypersensitivity is supported by the fact that insulin is well suited by its molecular characteristics for this type of immune reactions, and that the susceptible state of the organism allows this form of reaction to develop through subcutaneous injections. Apart from the clinical interest in the pathogenesis of this form of insulin allergy, an explanation on purely theoretical grounds would be very welcome. The causal relationship between delayed hypersensitivity and antibody production has long been discussed. These studies have been performed mainly in experimental animals. Therefore it would appear fruitful to investigate the immune reactions against insulin not only from the aspect of humoral antibodies, but also from that of delayed allergy.

2. Cytological Investigations

a) Immunofluorescence

α) The Different Techniques of Immunofluorescence

In immunofluorescence various methods are distinguished for the proof of an antigen or antibody on cells or in tissue: direct and indirect fluorescence, as well as the so-called "sandwich" technique.

In direct immunofluorescence, the tissue is first covered with a layer of labelled antibody or antigen, then freed from the uncombined agent by several washings, and finally mounted with a coverslip.

In indirect immunofluorescence, in the first step of the procedure, the characterizing antibody is not labelled but is stained in the second step by another antibody which is labelled, and directed against the first antibody.

Also in the sandwich technique the tissue requires double incubation. In contrast to indirect fluorescence, only one antibody is used, i. e. unlabelled antigen plus a labelled antibody identical to the antibody present in the tissue (for further details, see NAIRN, 1964).

For the investigation here planned the question is: how can insulin-sensitized cells and the cells producing antibodies against insulin be demonstrated by immunofluorescent methods? Direct immunofluorescence (layering of the cells with FITC-insulin = Fluorescein-Iso-Thio-Cyanate (= FITC) labelled insulin) is selected as the answer. The sandwich technique (layering of the cells with unmarked insulin and finally with an FITC-marked antibody) proved to be unsuitable. The reason for the failure of this technique, observed also by PARKER, ELEVITCH and GRODSKY (1963) is dealt within more detail on page 138.

β) Principles of Labelling with Fluorochromes

Fluorochromes contain certain reactive groups which will bind them to proteins; this is a real chief-valence binding, which guarantees a firm bond with the marker substance (v. MAYERSBACH, 1966). According to HOPKINS and WORMALL (1933), the $-N=C=S$ group reacts with aromatic amines, e. g. fluorescein isothiocyanate with the e-amino group of lysine.

According to TIETZE, MORTIMORE and LOMAX (1962), the fluorescein isothiocyanate is preferentially bound to phenylalanine of the B-chain, while an additional substitution on the terminal glycine portion can also occur. ARQUILLA, OOMS and FINN (1966) confirmed this.

The successful binding of protein with dye takes place in alkaline media, in the cold, where slow addition of the fluorochrome to the protein solution over 24 hours, with slow stirring, is advised (details see COONS and KAPLAN, 1950; MAYERSBACH, 1958, 1966; FOTHERGILL, 1964 a).

An essential simplification and enhancement of the marking stages was introduced by RINDERKNECHT (1960, 1962). The fluorochrome is absorbed onto Celite (a diatomaceous earth) whose large surface area provides generous dye-molecule binding. The dye molecules react rapidly with the protein without the need for an organic solvent, so that the protein can be added directly. However, not all proteins are marked to an equal extent (RINDERKNECHT, 1962), although these methods offer the great advantage of rapid and simple marking which is an essential condition for a good dye bond, according to CHADWICK et al. (1958 a, b) and PEARSE (1960). The marking method of COONS and KAPLAN and that of RINDERKNECHT have been applied to the following investigations.

γ) The Biologic Characteristics of FITC Insulin

The initial investigations of HALIKIS and ARQUILLA (1961) had shown that FITC-labelled insulin had a clearly reduced glucose-lowering effect (approximately 70%) in comparison to the active hormone. This percentage of effectiveness is not to be taken as absolute, since higher doses gave a relatively greater blood sugar reduction. TIETZE, MORTIMORE and LOMAX (1962) tested the insulin activity on guinea pigs and found only a 20% reduction of the glucose-lowering effect. Finally, ARQUILLA, OOMS and FINN (1966) reported that they observed a complete preservation of the biologic activity of FITC insulin, as against unlabelled insulin, when the FITC insulin was purified by means of acrylamide gel electrophoresis.

The FITC insulin employed in these investigations had 87% biologic activity (blood sugar reduction in rabbits), compared with an equal dose of unlabelled hormone (MAGER, 1966). It moved as a uniform band in the electrophoresis.

δ) The Immunological Characteristics of FITC Insulin

The immunological effectiveness of FITC-labelled insulin is considerably more important to these investigations than its biological activity.

The addition of a dye molecule could produce a diminution (or intensification?) of the immunologic characteristics through its influence upon the antigenic determinants. HALIKIS and ARQUILLA (1961) found that sheep erythrocytes, labelled with FITC insulin, agglutinated only in the initial dilutions, i. e. in the higher antibody

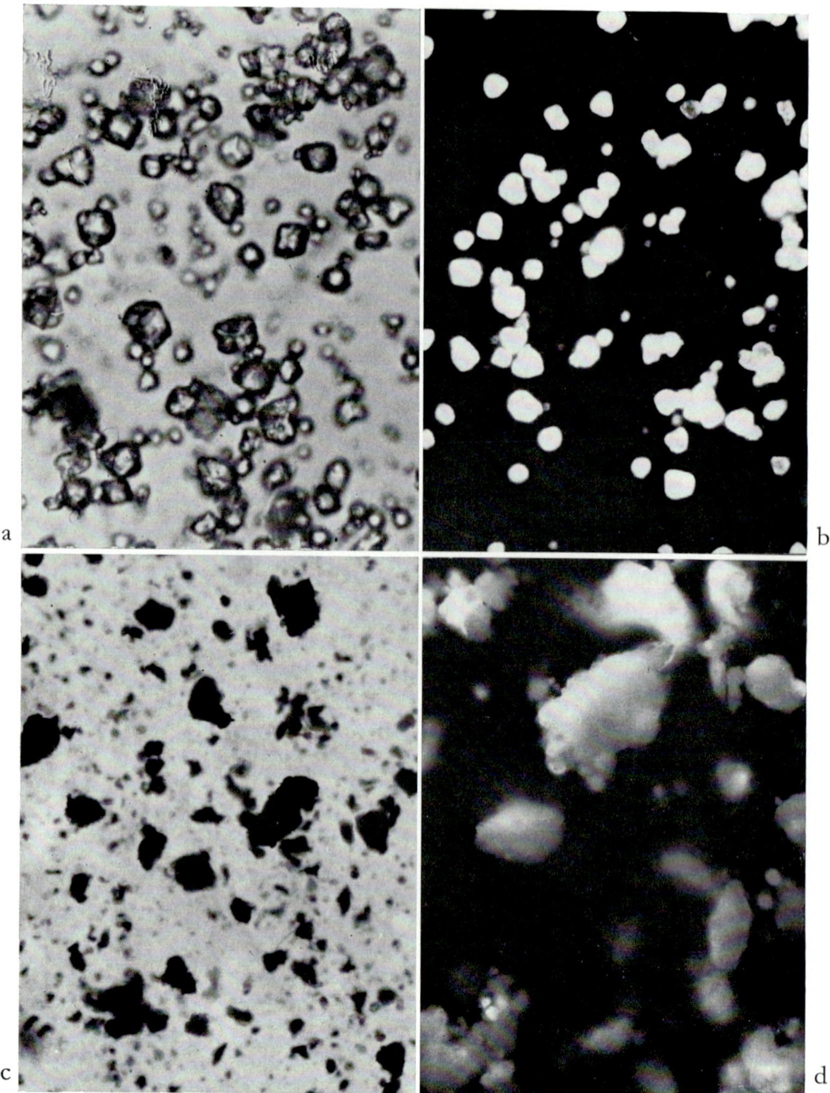

Fig. 4. FITC labelled insulin (bovine). a—b with a low F/P-ratio (*F*luorochrome/*P*rotein-ratio), optimally coupled insulin which retains the crystalline structure of insulin; c—d with a high F/P-ratio, overcoupled insulin, which has lost its crystalline structure and appears as amorphous powder. a and c Normal microscopical light; b and d Ultraviolet light (fluorescence microscope)

concentrations. However, FITC insulin in solution showed no alteration of its activity with antibody in comparison to unlabelled insulin. The diminution of immunological activity appeared to be linked to the technique of labelling the sheep erythrocytes with FITC insulin. More exact conclusions of the extent of this influence upon the antigenic determinants of the insulin molecule could not be reached.

More recent investigations by this group (ARQUILLA, OOMS and FINN, 1966) indicated that FITC insulin, purified by acrylamide gel electrophoresis, had the same immunological characteristics as unlabelled crystalline insulin. Both substances were then tested for their ability to limit immune hemolysis.

It is quite probable that the initial investigations of these authors were carried out with insulin which had been "overconjugated", i. e. either each molecule contained an excess of dye molecules, or far too many insulin molecules had been labelled. As MAGER (1966) found, crystallized FITC insulin is in all appearances identical to normal insulin if the molar dye/protein ratio is not too large, otherwise it consists of an amorphous powder (see Fig. 4).

The FITC insulin employed in the present work had a molar dye/protein ratio of 0.07 about 0,1. It is theoretically possible that some insulin molecules bore more than one dye molecule, but this has no effect on the preponderance of monosubstituted molecules.

ε) The Conjugation of Insulin with FITC

Pure insulin 500 mg is dissolved at 0° C in 6 ml of 0.5 M carbonate buffer ($Na_2CO_3 + NaHCO_3$) whose pH is 9.0. The insulin solution is diluted with 21 ml of 0.15 M NaCl to form an 0.87% solution. Then to the solution 4.2 ml Dioxan and 0.4 ml acetone is added, and the mixture is vigorously stirred. During cooling in the icebath, 1.5 ml of a 2% solution of fluorescein isothiocyanate (Fluka Company) is added dropwise, and the solution is simultaneously stirred vigorously. After continuous stirring overnight at 0°, the solution is adjusted to a pH of 5.2 by addition of HCl, and the reaction

* The conjugation was carried out by Dr. A. MAGER (Hoechst Company) according to the methods of POETSCHKE et al. (1957). Recrystallization is done according to the method of Hoechst Company. We take this opportunity to express our gratitude for the service rendered by Dr. MAGER and the Hoechst Company.

product is isoelectrically precipitated. The precipitated material is desiccated with acetone ether and subsequently crystallized. By repeated recrystallizations the overcoupled insulin is removed.

ζ) The Conjugation of Insulin Antibodies with FITC

The globulin fraction is precipitated out of guinea pig immune serum by saturated ammonium sulfate solution, or the 7 S globulin fraction is isolated by means of a DEAE Sephadex-A 50 column chromatography.

Subsequently the determination is made of the protein concentration of the solution which is then diluted with an equal volume of 0.5 M sodium carbonate-bicarbonate buffer whose pH is 9.0. Then FITC on Celite (Calbiochem, Los Angeles) is given in a quantity corresponding to 0.25 mg dye to 1 mg protein. The protein-dye mixture is cautiously shaken for 30 minutes and then centrifuged for 3 minutes at 1000 rpm. The supernatant is freed of unbound dye via Sephadex G 25 (4 gm Sephadex G 25 fine steeped overnight in 0.05 M sodium phosphate buffer, pH 6.5). Should a dilution occur during the chromatography, the labelled protein solution can be reconstituted by means of Carbowax (mol wt. 20,000). The labelled antibody is preserved by the addition of a few drops of a 1 : 20 solution of 1% Cialit (Asid, Munich). The reactive capacity of the antibody is tested with fresh rat pancreas (frozen section) or with passive hemagglutination. The molar dye/protein relationship (d/p ratio) is always between 1 and 1.5 for the antibodies employed.

η) The Isolation of Blood Leucocytes

For the isolation of white blood cells 0.1 ml of heparin (Liquemin, Roche) is added to 10 ml whole blood. After erythrocyte sedimentation the plasma is pipetted out. The quantity thus obtained (according to the sedimentation rate of the erythrocytes), approximately 1—4 ml, is made up to 10 ml by the addition of a citrate-saline solution (one part 3.8% Na citrate to 9 parts physiologic saline), and centrifuged in the cooled centrifuge at 1000 rpm for 4 minutes to free the cells from the plasma components. This stage is repeated three times. The washed sediment in a given quantity of saline-citrate solution reaches a concentration of 6×10^6 cells/mm³. Subsequently 0.1 ml of a 0.1 M $MgCl_2$ solution is given for each ml of leukocyte suspension.

From this cell suspension, 0.5 ml is pipetted onto the center of a siliconized slide, to permit spreading of the leukocytes over the glass surface. The slides are placed in a Petri dish and placed in an incubator at 37° C.*

The siliconization of the slides is performed as follows: the slides are cleaned with ether and then submerged for a few seconds in a 2% solution of silicon oil. After the excess fluid has drained off, the slides are glazed at 300° C for four hours to achieve a thin film.

After sedimentation of the leukocytes, the supernatant is pipetted off and the slide is air-dried for three minutes. Then the cells are incubated with FITC insulin.

ϑ) Separation of Lymphocytes and Granulocytes

For the separation of leukocytes into granulocytes and lymphocytes, the method of RABINOWITZ (1964), based on the investigations of GARVIN (1961), was employed.

Principle. A suspension of leukocytes is pipetted onto a column of the smallest siliconized glass pearls, which are enclosed in a heated water mantle (37° C). At 37° C the granulocytes spread over the glass pearls, owing to their adhesiveness. The lymphocytes can be simply washed out. Subsequently the granulocytes can be resuspended in ethylenediamine tetracetic acid (EDTA), and thereby recovered in isolation. (Fig. 5).

This method gives nearly pure lymphocyte and granulocyte suspensions (Figs. 6 and 7).

Technique. 40 ml of heparinized blood (1 : 100) is allowed to stand in a 10 ml glass tube at room temperature or at 4° C in a refrigerator (at a slower sedimentation rate) until enough plasma has separated from the erythrocytes, and may be pipetted off. The blood is then centrifuged in the cooled centrifuge for 4 minutes at 1400 rpm to separate the plasma supernant from the cell sediment. The cells are then resuspended in 3.5 ml plasma; the remaining plasma is put aside.

The plasma cell suspension is carefully transferred via a Record syringe through the rubber stopper of the glass vial into the glass pearls until the contents of the syringe have been distributed drop by drop into the column (there should be approx. 1 cm of free space

* Priv. Doz. Dr. K. BREDDIN is herewith thanked for his proposals for cell recovery.

in the column above the pearls). Then the column is held at 37° C for 30 minutes to effect adhesion of the granulocytes and monocytes.

Meanwhile the retained plasma is completely freed of cells by centrifugation in the cooled centrifuge for 10 minutes at 7000 rpm.

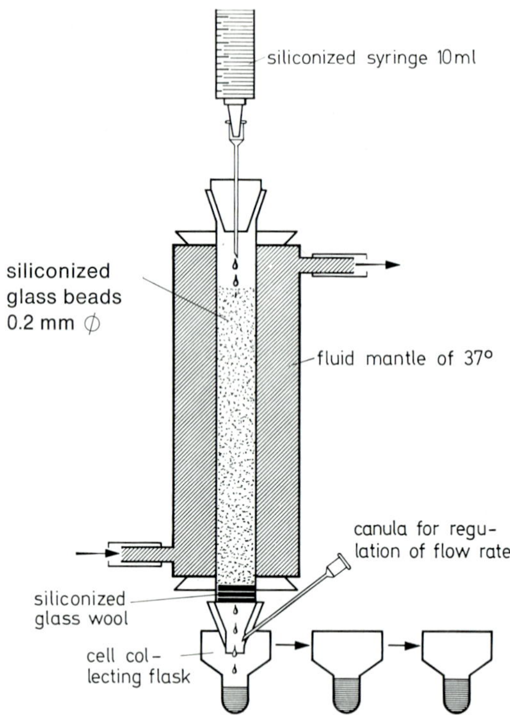

Fig. 5. Scheme of a glass bead column for separation of blood lymphocytes and granulocytes (according to RABINOWITZ, 1964)

At the end of the column incubation period, the non-adhering cells (lymphocytes and a few erythrocytes) are washed out of the column by 4 ml of the cell-free plasma. These form the first fraction. Then the remaining non-adhering cells are washed out by the drop-wise instillation of 30 ml Hanks Solution from an Erlenmeyer flask. This washing fluid is discarded.

The granulocytes and monocytes are obtained by washing the column with 40 ml of a 0.2% solution of EDTA. The run-off contains

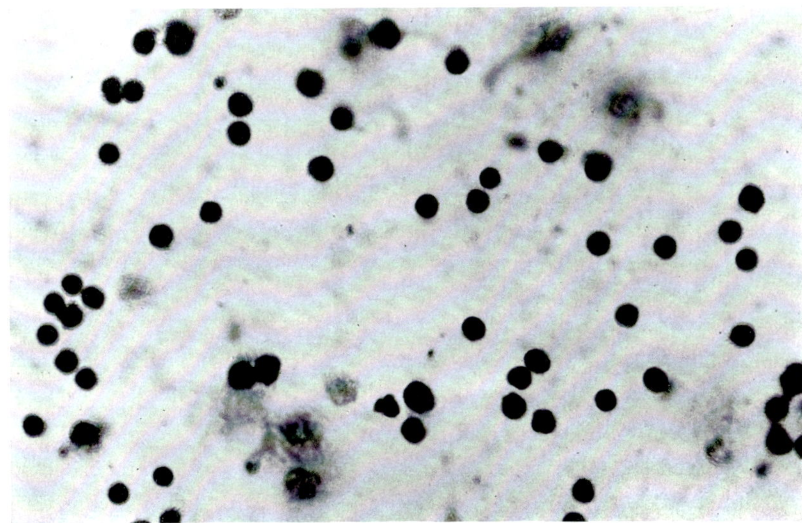

Fig. 6. Fraction of isolated blood lymphocytes. Pappenheim staining. ×550

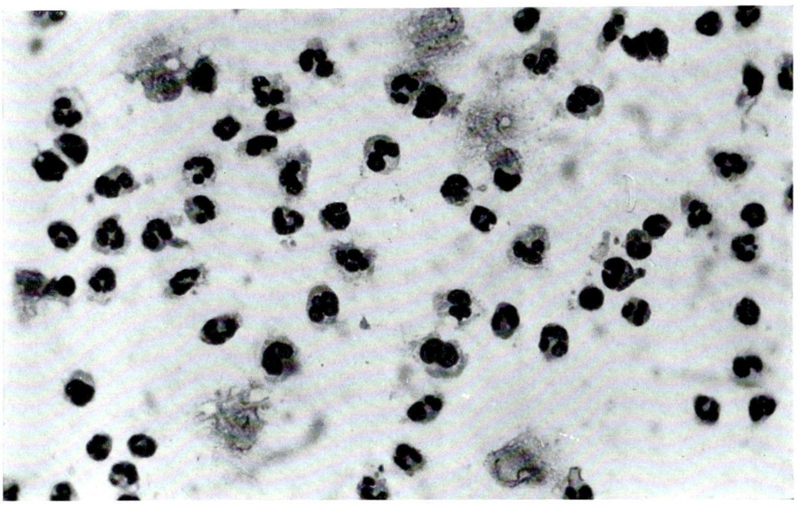

Fig. 7. Fraction of isolated blood granulocytes. Pappenheim staining. ×550

the second fraction, in which the first portion consists of granulocytes and the latter of monocytes. The subsequent cell processing up to the incubation with FITC insulin is described on pp. 37.

ι) *The Application of Immunofluorescence to Blood Cells*

10 mg FITC insulin are dissolved in 3 ml aqua dest.; the slightly cloudy solution is made clear by "Hanks balanced salt solution" from Difco Bacto Laboratories, Detroit, Michigan, U.S.A., stirring with a glass rod wetted with 1 N HCl. The solution is diluted in a 1 : 5 proportion with isotonic phosphate buffer (pH 7.5). 0.1 ml of this dilute solution is layered over the cell preparation and incubated at 37° C for 30 minutes. Subsequently the unbound insulin is carefully washed away with Mayer's Buffer (pH 7.5), the slide is washed in a cuvette with Mayer's Buffer for over 10 minutes, and finally covered with a mixture of Mayer's Buffer and glycerin in a proportion of 3 : 1. To prevent dehydration of the specimens, they are encased in warm beeswax.

The sandwich technique, employed initially but later discarded due to lack of specificity, was carried out thus: incubation of the blood cells with unlabelled insulin in the same manner as with FITC insulin (see above) for 30 minutes at 37° C; then washing for 10 minutes with Mayer's Buffer; repeat incubation for 30 minutes at 37° C with an FITC anti-insulin antibody; then 10 minutes' washing and subsequent covering with Mayer's Buffer as above.

κ) *Specificity Tests for Immunofluorescence*

The cell-bound antibody against insulin, as well as the anti-insulin antibody produced in plasma cells or in their precursors, is demonstrable by direct immunofluorescence (incubation with FITC-labelled insulin).

The following specificity tests were employed:

1. Inhibition test: Prior incubation with unlabelled insulin to saturate the antigen-binding sites. Then incubation with labelled insulin. A specific reaction must fail to occur or at least be very slight.

2. Test with a nonspecific antigen: incubation with FITC-labelled bovine serum albumin (BSA). There must be no binding of this material by the sensitized cells.

3. The specimens were incubated with free dye (FITC).

4. Test with the unsensitized cells of a normal person: no binding of FITC-insulin should occur, due to lack of antigen-binding sites.

Investigations were made of leukocyte preparations from the blood of patients with eosinophilia (ascaridiasis and reticulosis) to determine their binding capacity for FITC insulin and free dye. v. MAYERSBACH (1966) and v. MAYERSBACH and SCHUBERT (1960) have described the ability of eosinophils in blood and tissue to bind acid dyes which is a prime reason for nonspecific dye fixation.

As a check on binding by immunofluorescence, another method was employed which rests on a quite different basis, i. e. one which does not involve a dye technique. This is discussed under Immune Adherence. (C.I.2.b)

λ) The Evaluation of the Cytologic Preparations

Blood leukocyte preparations (total leukocytes or various kinds) are made up with varying cell density for mounting on glass slides. Only those preparations were evaluated which had sufficient density, yet permitted identification of single cells. A weak unspecific dye uptake by the non-reactive cells is necessary for their identification. By dividing the optical field with crossed lines in the ocular lens, one is able to count 500 cells pro field and enumerate them in a cell counter (Ferrari-Statitest). The number of specifically fluorescing cells is given as a percentage.

b) Immune Adherence

α) Introductory Remarks

Apart from the specificity test of immuno-fluorescence, the bind ing of insulin to immunologically active cells (whether actively or passively sensitized) is demonstrable by other methods employing different principles. The most suitable technique appeared to be one enabling the reaction between white blood cells and the antigen to be demonstrated using erythrocytes as indicators — the immuno-cyto-adherence test of NOTA, LIACOPOULOS-BRIOT, STIFFEL and BIOZZI (1964) or the immune adherence test of NELSON (1953). The predictability of this test will be discussed later. Suffice it to say that both techniques can provide evidence both of humoral antibodies and of the presence of delayed hypersensitivity (sensitized cells). NOTA et al. employ their technique for the proof of antibody-forming cells (i. e.

the demonstration of humoral antibodies), while COOMBS and GELL (1968) have employed their method as one of the few approaches to the demonstration of delayed allergy. But NELSON's immune adherence test is recognized as sensitive and very specific as evidence of circulating antibodies, while others have used it to demonstrate sensitized lymphocytes (FUJI and NELSON, 1963). Both techniques utilize erythrocytes as the reaction indicator. There are, however, important general differences. According to NOTA et al., the antigen is bound to the erythrocyte which then reacts with the immunologically competent cells. The reaction proceeds in the absence of complement. However, the immune adherence test involves a reaction between antibody and antigen (here, between immunologically active cells and insulin). To form the antigen-antibody complex, complement is added to the reaction mixture. The last agents for the reaction are the Group 0 erythrocytes (Rh+) which specifically adhere to the antigen-antibody-complement complex. The advantage of this technique over that of NOTA et al. is that all the components of the reaction are able to work on each other in exactly calculable concentrations, while the quantity (concentration) of antigen passively bound to the erythrocyte is always subject to variation.

β) Technique

The white blood cells are washed three times in isotonic phosphate buffer (pH 7.5), and are concentrated in a quantity of 1×10^6/ml. For this reaction the following mixture is required:

a) Guinea-pig complement, which is absorbed three times with a pool of leukocytes and erythrocytes of normal persons (controls) to eliminate any natural antibodies against human blood cells which may be present;

b) Insulin in a dilution of 1 mg/ml isotonic phosphate buffer;

c) Human erythrocytes (Group 0, Rh+) which have been washed three times in Mayer's Buffer with EDTA (final concentration of the buffer 0.01 M).

0.25 ml of the leukocyte suspension, 0.1 ml insulin and 0.1 ml complement (diluted 1 : 10 in tyrode solution) are incubated together for one hour at 37° C and simultaneously shaken. Then 0.1 ml of the erythrocyte suspension (in a concentration of 1×10^7/ml) is added, and the mixture is incubated with shaking, as above. Small drops of this mixture are placed on glass slides and covered with a coverslip. The microscopic evaluation is performed using phase contrast.

γ) *Specificity Tests for Immune Adherence*

In specificity tests the leukocytes (all leukocytes or specific kinds) are incubated and finally evaluated with:

erythrocytes and insulin (without complement)
erythrocytes and complement (without insulin)
erythrocytes (without insulin and without complement).

A further check is evaluation of the leukocytes of normal persons.

δ) *The Evaluation of Cytologic Preparations*

From every blood test (using all leukocytes or specific kinds) 500 cells are counted, and those with one or more adherent erythrocytes are scored as positive (corresponding to the method of FUJI and NELSON, 1963). An accidental accumulation is ruled out by mechanical pressure upon the preparation. Immune adherent erythrocytes are not detached from the leukocytes.

c) *Lymphocyte Transformation*

α) *Introductory Remarks*

As a further method of identifying insulin-sensitized cells in the blood of patients with insulin allergy, in vitro lymphocyte transformation is employed. In 1960, NOWELL discovered that human lymphocytes (from blood) undergo an in vitro transformation into blast-like forms when phytohemagglutinin (PHA) is added to the culture medium. In 1963 PEARMAIN, LYSETTE and FITZGERALD found that the same effect is achieved by cultivating the leukocytes of tuberculin-sensitive individuals with the specific antigen, i. g. tuberculin. Later it was shown that lymphocyte stimulation also occurred in the immediate allergy category, i. e. pollen allergy (ZEITZ, VAN ARSDEL and MCCLURE, 1966), as well as in the delayed allergy category. HALPERN, KY and AMACHE (1967) have been able to demonstrate increased lymphocyte transformation in the immediate response to insulin of patients who had experienced generalized urticaria after insulin. The delayed response to insulin was initially demonstrated by the work of our own group (FEDERLIN, KRIEGBAUM and FLAD, 1968).

β) Technique

20 ml of blood is obtained in a disposable syringe containing 3 drops of heparin (Liquemin; Roche). Sedimentation of the erythrocytes is accomplished by inverting the syringe to the vertical position for 45 min. at 37° C. The plasma is drawn off through a no. 1 needle into another 20 ml disposable syringe which is packed with nylon fibers. The plasma should stand in this syringe for 45 min. at 37° C. (The granulocytes become attached to the nylon fibers). The packing is washed with the culture medium (TC 199 or Eagle Medium L) until the rinse is clear. The rinses are collected in sterile 5—6 ml tubes and centrifuged at 1000 rpm for 10 minutes. The sediment is washed with 5 ml of culture medium and again centrifuged. The sediment is resuspended in 1 ml of culture medium, smeared on glass slides and stained (Pappenheim). The cell concentration of the suspension is determined in a Neubauer counting chamber. The cell suspension is diluted to 1×10^6 cells/ml culture medium (the culture medium consists of: 80% Eagle L Medium; 20% calf serum without complement; penicillin 100 units + streptomycin 100 µg/ml). Antigen components 50 to 500 µg insulin/ml. Phytohemagglutinin component 0.01—0.1 ml. Duration of incubation: PHA stimulation 72 hrs; antigen-stimulation 120 hrs. Total quantity (incl. medium) per tube: 3 ml. Incubation temperature: 37 °C.

Harvesting the cultures: the culture medium is carefully pipetted out, the cells are stirred wih a fine Pasteur pipette and a 3 : 1 solution of methanol and glacial acetic acid is added. Fixation requires 10 min.

Then the suspension is centrifuged for 5 minutes. The sediment and remaining fixative is added dropwise to glass slides, and then stained (Pappenheim technique: 1 min. May-Grünwald sol.; Giemsa sol. 20 min. The concentrated Giemsa solution is diluted 1 : 20 with Sörensen buffer).

γ) Evaluation of the Cell Preparations

To assess the extent of lymphocyte transformation due to antigenic stimulation, the preparations of the various culture groups are thus arranged:

a) Lymphocytes after culturing in medium alone
b) Lymphocytes after culturing with PHA
c) Lymphocytes after culturing with antigen.

500 cells are counted, and the number of transformed cells is given as a percentage.

d) The Cytology of the Peripheric Blood Cells

A panoptic staining was performed for the morphological identification of the white blood cell preparations on siliconized slides (Pappenheim staining). The air-dried sedimented cells were fixed for one minute with May-Grünwald solution. The solution was diluted in addition with a few ml of distilled water for two minutes. After rinsing with distilled water, the specimens were counterstained for 20 minutes with a Giemsa solution (diluted 1 : 20 in distilled water). The dried preparations were covered with Eukitt. By means of a cell counter (Ferrari-Statitest) 200 cells of each preparation were counted.

The purpose of these examinations was to compare the shape of the cells on siliconized slides with those of normal slides and to obtain information about the number of eosinophils.

3. The Intracutaneous Skin Test

An intracutaneous skin test was carried out on all patients with various insulin preparations. Thus, 0.02 ml of an insulin solution, diluted with physiological saline to an end concentration of 2 units/ml, was injected intracutaneously through the finest needle available (no. 20). In the same dilution, the pharmacologic co-substances Surfen, Chloraeton, Solbrol and "Lente" were prepared and tested.

4. Histological and Immunofluorescent Studies in Skin Biopsies

Patients with the clinical picture of delayed skin allergy to insulin had excisional skin biopsies * and these were examined both histologically and immunologically (author). The excised skin was divided lengthwise immediately after being obtained. One half was fixed in formalin, then embedded in paraffin wax in the Autotechnicon via methylbenzoate. Staining utilized haematoxylin-eosin and Giemsa. The other half was immediately deep-frozen and then sectioned in the cryostat (Dittes-Duspiva system). The unfixed sections were

---

* I am grateful to Professor STÜTTGEN, formerly Department of Dermatology, University of Frankfurt/Main, for carrying out the skin biopsies and the histological evaluation.

evaluated immunohistologically for insulin antibodies and for any antigen still present. These investigations were accomplished using the technique described on page 40.

5. Investigations of Humoral Insulin Antibodies

Together with the investigations of sensitized cells, all test sera were evaluated for the presence of humoral anti-insulin antibodies. This was done for various reasons: it should be investigated whether the stage of a delayed immune reaction precedes the production of humoral antibodies; furthermore, the humoral antibodies could be present as both neutralizing and skin-sensitizing antibodies. The two forms had to be investigated by different techniques, apart from the fact that their manifestations are different. Thus the essential question for delayed insulin allergy is this: are all cutaneous reactions to insulin associated to some extent with certain humoral antibodies? Not all cases present clearly enough in their clinical manifestation to allow a delayed immune response to insulin to be distinguished from a possible delayed early (i. e. immediate) reaction. Occasionally it is difficult to differentiate clearly (MARBLE, 1959 a, b), although it is likely that quite different pathogenic mechanisms underlie the clinical phenomena.

There is also the problem of the so-called cytophilic antibody (BOYDEN and SORKIN, 1963). This is a globulin component which can be absorbed by different cell types, so that they then react specifically with the corresponding antigen. Even cells of a non-immunized animal can be sensitized. The authors suggested that these cytophilic antibodies play a role in immune reactions of the delayed type. Cytophilic antibodies have so far only been found in certain species (in the sera of guinea pigs, horses and rabbits), although only a few antigens have been evaluated for this characteristic. Insulin was not among these antigens. Most interestingly, however, ROSE and BROWN (1962) demonstrated cytophilic antibody against another hormonal substance, thyroglobulin. The fixation capacity of this type of antibody has been shown in various rabbit tissues, as well as in granulocytes from the peritoneal cavity and from the bone marrow (BOYDEN and SORKIN, 1960, 1961). The question arises whether certain cytophilic antibodies are responsible for the reaction of blood cells with the antigen insulin.

For the determination of neutralizing antibodies against insulin, the insulin-binding capacity for ^{131}I insulin is evaluated according to the methods of BERSON and YALOW (1959 a). And as a purely immunologic method, the passive hemagglutinin method of ARQUILLA and STAVITSKY (1956 a, b) is also performed.

a) Insulin-Neutralizing Antibodies

α) Measurement of Maximum Insulin-binding Capacity

Principle. Measured quantities of radioactively labelled and unlabelled insulin are added to varied dilutions of serum. The mixture is kept at 4° C for three days, so that both sites of the insulin molecule can compete for the binding site of the antibody contained in the serum. Then an ion-exchange substance, Amberlite, is employed, which removes the antibody with its bound insulin from the solution. After sedimentation, the radioactivity of the supernatant is measured and hence the concentration of the unbound, labelled insulin.

The calculation of the maximum binding capacity of the individual serum dilutions is made graphically from the ratio of free to bound ^{131}iodine insulin and the corresponding quantity of bound insulin, according to the instructions of BERSON and YALOW (1959 a). The author is very grateful to Dr. J. D. FAULHABER and Prof. H. DITSCHUNEIT for assistance in the measurement of some sera.

(For further technical details regarding the measurement of insulin antibodies see KERP, STEINHILBER and KASEMIR, 1966; DITSCHUNEIT and FEDERLIN, 1966; PFEIFFER, DITSCHUNEIT and FEDERLIN, 1969).

Method. 0.5 ml of standard insulin (bovine insulin, 1 mg = 27.5 U) is made up to varying end concentrations (0—500—2000—10 000—100 000 μU/ml) and mixed with 0.5 ml ^{131}I-insulin in an end concentration of 1—2 μU/ml, and with 0.01 ml and 0.001 ml of the sera to be tested. These preparations are kept at 4° C for 3 days. Then 100 mg Amberlite (Type CG 400 I in OH form) is added to each, and the solutions are well shaken for 20—30 minutes. After sedimentation of the Amberlite, the radioactivity of portions of 0.1 and of 0.2 ml of the supernatant is measured by a liquid scintillation counter.

β) Passive Hemagglutination

Principle. BOYDEN (1951) initially recognized the possibility of binding proteins to erythrocytes which had been pretreated with tannic acid. The cells could be made to take up the antigen, and then to agglutinate after the addition of the corresponding antibody. This process was inhibited by the pre-incubation of antibody with antigen. The addition of complement creates a hemolytic system and the extent of hemolysis can be measured. A different technique using bisdiazobenzidine binds the proteins to erythrocytes as in azo compounds. The technique is described by PRESSMAN, CAMPBELL and PAULING (1942). It has the advantage that no hemolysis occurs, and also that the bond between the antigen and the erythrocyte surface seems to be firmer.

Methods. Rabbit erythrocytes are drawn up in a 1 : 1 ratio in Alsever's Solution and washed three times with Alsever's Solution. *

2. Rabbit normal serum (RNS) and antiserum are heated at 56° C for 30 minutes to remove complement; the RNS is then diluted 1 : 100 in physiological saline.

3. A dilutional sequence of RNS from 1 : 10 to 1 : 196,830 (10 tubes) is set up.

In the first tube 0.45 ml diluted RNS

In the 2nd—10th tubes 0.50 ml diluted RNS.

4. The antiserum without complement is absorbed on rabbit erythrocytes (20 parts serum + 1 part rabbit erythrocytes); the suspension is kept in an ice bath with occasional shaking. Then the suspension is centrifuged at the highest speed and decanted.

5. 0.05 ml of the antiserum, already absorbed and freed of complement, is pipetted into the first tube of dilutional sequence and thereafter 0.25 ml to each tube of the sequence through to the last.

6. The coupling of the antigen onto the erythrocyte:

6 mg insulin is dissolved in 1 ml n/300 HCl. Then 5.0 ml of isotonic phosphate buffer and 3.0 ml of physiological saline are added. After complete mixing, 0.2 ml of washed rabbit erythrocytes is added.

7. 1.5 mg bisdiazobenzidine is carefully dissolved in 19.75 ml of isotonic phosphate buffer; erythrocytes are added slowly. The suspension is left standing at room temperature for 10 minutes, with occasional gentle shaking. Then the suspension is centrifuged for

* Alsever's Solution
2.05 gm dextrose
0.8 gm Na citrate
042 gm NaCl
aqua dist. to 100 ml, pH regulation to 6.1 with 10% citric acid.

5 minutes at 2000 rpm. The erythrocytes are washed three times with RNS, and finally suspended in thrice diluted RNS.

8. 0.05 ml of the erythrocyte suspension is pipetted into every tube of the previously prepared dilutional sequence and the mixture is well shaken. They are left to stand for 3 h before being read.

Control

1. For every run, the antiserum is diluted 1 : 10 and mixed in the usual manner with 0.05 ml of already bound erythrocytes.

2. A complete dilutional sequence is set up with antisera, to which is added 0.05 ml of unbound erythrocytes. (3 ml RNS + 0.2 ml of the washed rabbit-erythrocytes sediment).

b) Skin-sensitizing Antibody (Reagin)

α) Remarks

The essential biological characteristic of reagins is their fixation on tissue cells of the skin, and mucosa in particular. They remain there, unlike all other antibodies, for weeks or months, and can also be demonstrated for a long time in control subjects after passive transfer. This characteristic is the basis of the test of PRAUSNITZ and KÜSTNER (1921) for the proof of reagins. A small amount of serum, which is presumed to contain the antibody, is injected intracutaneously into a healthy control subject. A small dose of antigen, injected 48 hours later into the same site, evokes a characteristic reaction with a central reddening and circumferential pallor. This is caused by the antigen-antibody reaction, which liberates such substances as histamine, serotonin, bradykinin, etc. Another characteristic of reagins is their inactivation by heating for several hours at 56° C. A minimum of 30 minutes and a maximum of 10 hours are necessary. A serum thus treated will evoke no skin reaction, for which reason a specificity control of the P-K test must always be performed with inactivated serum.

This pioneer work has remained the single definite test for reagins up to now. However, the test has the great disadvantage that it must always be carried out on a normal human control subject, since all efforts to apply it to laboratory animals have failed. The ever-growing danger that the normal person may receive the virus of homologous serum hepatitis, even from clinically healthy persons, makes the technique of the P-K test ethically dubious.

Recently, LAYTON et al. (1962) were able to show that rhesus monkeys could be passively sensitized with human serum. The authors were able to demonstrate reagins against plant protein *(Ricinus communis)*. This was not, however, accomplished with the original PRAUSNITZ-KÜSTNER technique. They employed the passive cutaneous anaphylaxis technique (PCA) of OVARY (1958, 1959, 1964). According to this method, the test serum is injected into the skin of the back of guinea pigs. Three to four hours later, the presumed antigen, together with a dye, is injected intravenously. The subsequent reaction of the antigen with the antibody present in the tissue initiates a vascular alteration permitting the transport of dye into the nearby region, which is recognizable either from outside or from inside the dermis. By the quite sensitive method, antibody as well as antigen can be demonstrated.

The evidence that LAYTON et al. (1965) with PCA demonstrated a reagin and not a "normal" anaphylactic antibody of the 7-S type, is expressed by the fact that the reaction was still positive even 48 hours after the injection of the antibody. The maximum duration of fixation for other types of antibodies is usually between 24—48 hours (HUMPHREY and WHITE, 1964). A further proof was the negative result after inactivation of the serum by heating to 56° C.

This technique, described as the "allergic serum transfer test", consists of a mixture of the original Prausnitz-Küstner technique and the usual Ovary technique.

β) The "Allergic Serum Transfer Test" (AST Test)

Principle: The usual AST test proved to be unsuitable for indicating reagins against insulin in rhesus monkeys. Serious hypoglycemic shock after intravenous injection of the antigen insulin can only be avoided by using such small doses that a visible antigen-antibody reaction does not take place. To exclude these difficulties, biologically-inactive insulin * was employed.

The inactivation of the hormone is accomplished by treatment with a strong base which effects a breakdown of the –S–S bridge between the amino acids at positions 6 and 11 of the A chain. Large quantities of inactivated insulin can be injected intravenously without

* Dr. A. MAGER (Hoechst Company) is thanked for supplying this insulin.

signs of hypoglycemia. The "allergic serum transfer test", with this insulin, is positive; the dose corresponds to 20—40 units of active regular insulin.

Method. The investigation was carried out with rhesus monkeys (*Macacus rhesus*) of 3 kg weight. Dr. HEBER (veterinary surgeon, Paul Ehrlich Institute, Frankfurt a. M.) is thanked for his assistance. The animals were shaved over the body and proximal extremities. Those monkeys having the least number of blue spots were selected; this characteristic is very frequently observed in rhesus monkeys.

Into areas free from blue spots, 0.1 ml of the test serum was injected intracutaneously (abdominal wall, thigh, upper arm, eyelid). After 48 hours, 2.0 ml of a 0.5% Evans Blue dye solution (sterile) was injected intravenously. After the dye had distributed itself (approximately 5 minutes), the antigen (inactive insulin) was injected intravenously in a dose corresponding to 20—40 units of regular active insulin. The dose was prepared in this manner: 13 mg of inactive insulin is dissolved in 50 ml aqua dest. with a minute quantity of 1 N NaOH to complete the dissolving of any precipitated insulin. 10 ml of isotonic phosphate buffer (pH 7.5) is added. 1 ml of this solution corresponds to 40 units of the customary regular insulin.

The monkeys were not anesthetized, but were held by their keepers so that any diminution of the immunological reaction by the anesthetic agent could be avoided.

The following control procedures were undertaken:

a) with dye alone, i. e. without antigen
b) with inactivated serum (4 hours at 56° C)
c) with normal serum
d) with serum from non-allergic diabetics.

To exclude a reaction caused by insulin antibodies which do not belong to the group of reagins, passive cutaneous anaphylaxis was carried out in the usual way in guinea pigs with the sera in question. Four hours after the intracutaneous administration of the serum, dye and antigen are injected intravenously, as in the above-mentioned technique.

c) The Investigation of Cytophilic Antibodies

Principle. (see page 46).

Method. Leukocytes of a healthy control subject are incubated for 8 hours at +4° C with the serum of a patient who is known to have delayed insulin allergy. The cells are then washed four times with HANKS' solution, resuspended in this solution, sedimented onto siliconized glass slides, and incubated with FITC insulin in the manner described for immunofluorescence on page 40.

6. Results

a) Case Reports

Case History no. 1

M. G. 66-year-old female patient

1967: Diabetes mellitus developed after ileus surgery and was treated with tolbutamide. In July 1966 blood sugar was 300 mg⁰/₀ and urine sugar 100 gm/24 h. Insulin therapy was initiated four days after the first injection,

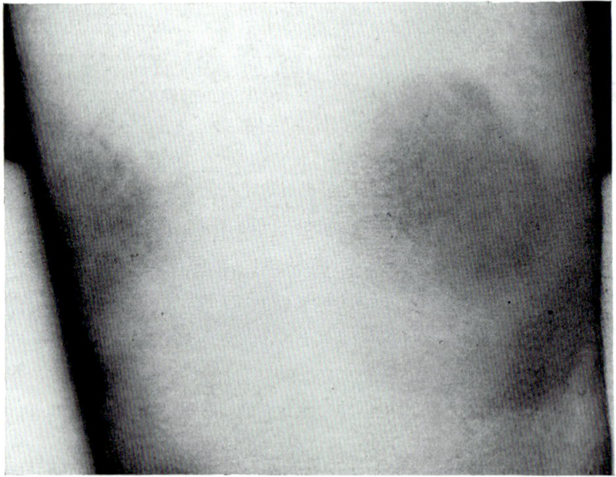

Fig. 8. Delayed allergic reaction (maximum 24—36 hours after the injection) to insulin on day 6 of treatment

a hard, painful erythema developed in the injection area; it was then 3 cm in diameter on the following days becoming palm-sized. The reaction occurred 8—10 hours after the injection, reaching a maximum size 24—26 hours after that. Insulin therapy was stopped and sulfonylurea maintainance began without improvement of the glucose metabolism. Administration of insulin was restarted with still greater skin reactions as a result. The patient was admitted to hospital with wood-hard induration (diameter approaching 7 cm — see Fig. 8) on both thighs. Clinical evaluation revealed no significant diagnostic finding. Leukocyte count was normal with a slight shift to the left; sedimentation rate 70; blood sugar 230 mg%; urine sugar 2 gm/24 hrs; skin test: strong delayed response to bovine insulin (after 24 hrs.); weak delayed response to porcine insulin no response to Surfen and the preservative Chloraeton (azetono-chloroform).

Immunocytology: before hospitalization, the immunofluorescent technique (incubation of white cells with FITC insulin) had shown 5% of cells with positive fluorescence. On admission, there was already a clearly increased number of antigen-binding leukocytes. There was particularly strong involvement of the lymphocytes (Figs. 9 and 10) approximately 60% at the time of the most intense skin reaction) and less of the granulocytes (Fig. 11) (maximum 17%). Note: this percentage of lymphocytes does not represent an absolute number, since during incubation with the antigen an unknown number of cells are washed from the slide.

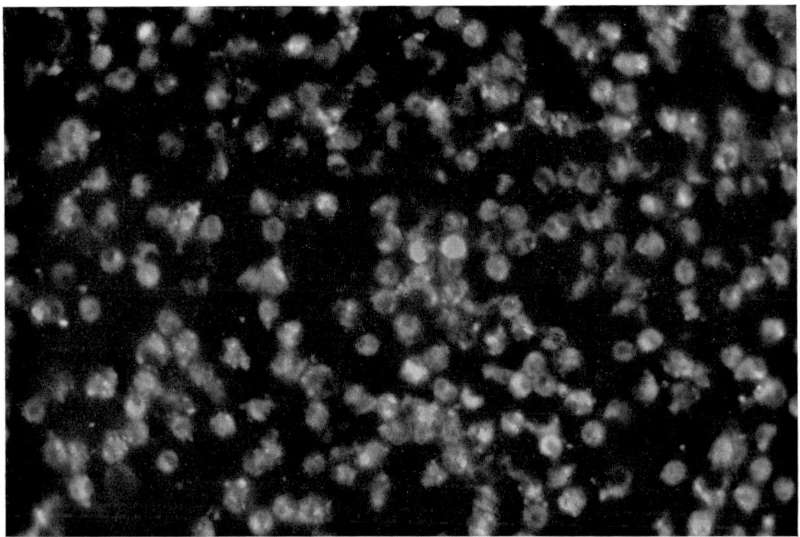

Fig. 9. White blood cells of a non-diabetic control after incubation with FITC-insulin. ×550

Further course: the degree of skin inflammation was so great that therapy was continued with pure porcine insulin (NOVO-Semilente). The skin manifestations regressed within a few days to only a minimal erythema, with a fall in the number of fluorescing cells (lymphocytes 12%, granulocytes 5%). During the following days, a delayed skin allergy to porcine insulin was seen, although to a small degree, with an increase in insulin-binding cells (lymphocytes 28%, granulocytes 20%). Investigation of serum antibodies showed maximum insulin-binding capacity (IBC) during the initial days of hospitalization — the time of the strong skin reaction — to

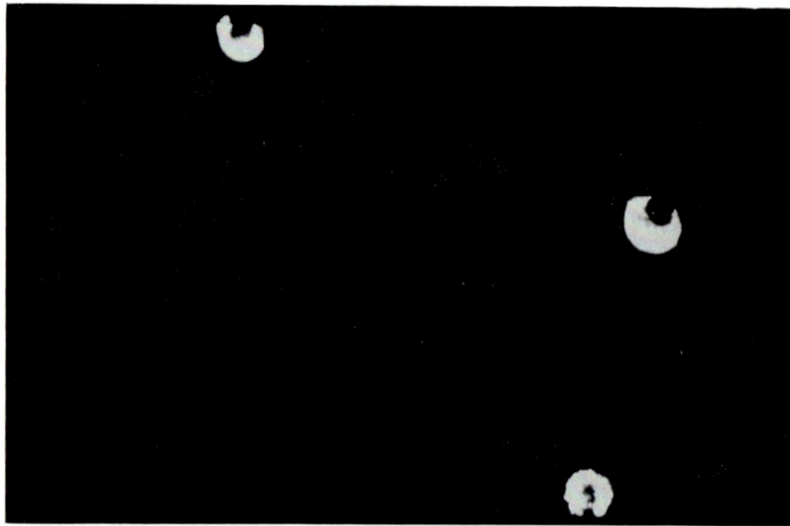

Fig. 10. Binding of FITC-insulin by lymphocytes of a patient with delayed insulin allergy. Immunofluorescence microscopy. ×1400

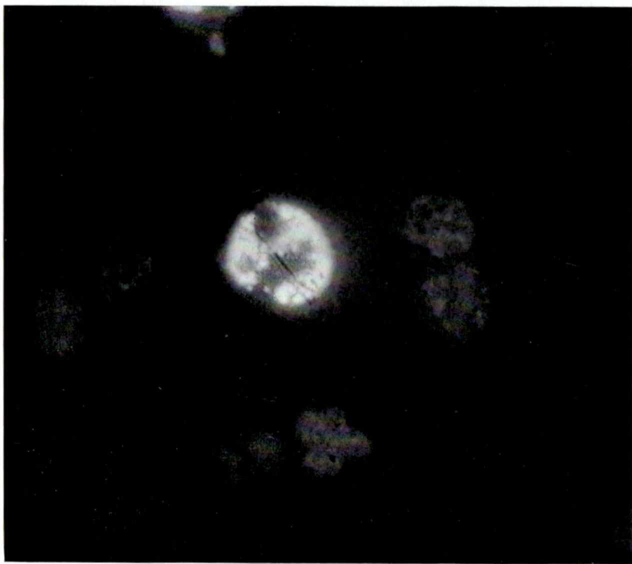

Fig. 11. Binding of FITC-insulin by granulocytes of a patient with long-lasting delayed allergy to insulin. ×1250

be 0.5 units/liter, i. e. normal. A few days later IBC had risen to 20 units and three weeks later to 101 units/liter. Passive hemagglutinin titer was 1 : 40. The investigation of skin-sensitizing antibodies (reagins) was negative.

Blood and urine sugar values remained effectively unchanged during these immunologic developments. The patient was discharged on 28 units Semilente (blood sugar 112 mg%, urine sugar 12 gm/24 hrs), still with mild delayed skin reaction. Again in the following months there was an increase in the allergy and in the insulin-binding cells (15—30% of all leukocytes), in the immunofluorescence and in the immune adherence (see Fig. 12). Because of increased reaction to porcine insulin, treatment was

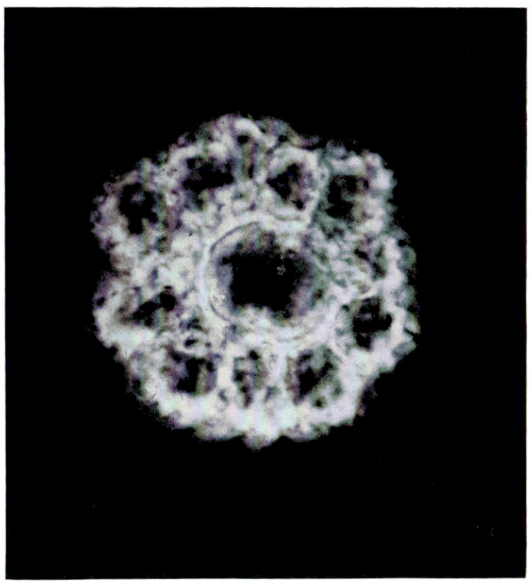

Fig. 12. Immune adherence. In center a lymphocyte of a patient with delayed insulin allergy, attachment of red cells of blood group 0 in presence of antigen and complement. ×1500

switched to bovine insulin; there was short-term regression of the skin manifestations, followed by an increase after four weeks. Sulfonylurea treatment was not possible. With mixed (bovine/porcine) insulin, satisfactory control of the diabetes was achieved despite mild skin reactions.

Discussion. This patient manifested a strong delayed allergy to bovine insulin, accompanied by marked antigen-binding by the sensitized leukocytes. Shortly after the onset of the delayed allergy, a humoral insulin-antibody of the neutralizing type developed to a maximal insulin-binding capacity of 100 units/liter. Transition to pure porcine insulin led to an extensive regression of the allergic reactions and to a decrease in the sensitized cells. However, within a few days a delayed allergy against this insulin developed, so that the treatment again was carried out with bovine insulin, which formerly appeared unsuccessful. After several months the delayed allergy to both types of insulin regressed gradually with continuing insulin therapy. Even the previously high concentration of insulin-binding antibody was eventually no longer observable. Apparently this represents a so-called desensitization, both for the delayed allergy and for the humoral antibodies.

Case History no. 2

I. S. 62-year-old female patient

1960: Diabetes mellitus was diagnosed and several week's insulin therapy was given. Treatment was changed to sulfonylureas until fall 1965. Following bronchitis with fever, this was changed to insulin. Seven days after the initiation of insulin injections (mixed bovine-porcine insulin), a delayed allergy developed at the injection site without affecting the glucose metabolism. Insulin therapy with porcine insulin was continued and there was a regression in the skin reaction but not complete resolution. The patient was therefore admitted to hospital.

On admission, 20 units Actrapid were being injected three times a day (blood sugar between 160—350 mg%, urine sugar 1—2 gm/24 hrs). In the region of the insulin injections there was an indurated area 3 cm in diameter, with maximum intensity 12 hours after injection. The skin test clearly showed a delayed allergy to bovine insulin, a weak reaction to porcine insulin, and a negative reaction to additive substances. The maximum immunofluorescence value of antigen-binding leukocytes was 14%; at the same time the maximum insulin-binding capacity of the serum was 40 units/liter. Under continued therapy with pure porcine insulin, a diminution of all allergic manifestations was observed.

Discussion. This patient represents a delayed cutaneous reaction, predominantly against bovine insulin, and only to a limited extent against porcine insulin; this allergy was already declining when the patient entered hospital. Humoral antibodies had already developed. Both types of immune mechanism coexisted at the time of observation. Spontaneous desensitization developed under continued therapy with porcine insulin.

Case History no. 3

E. T. 55-year-old female patient

In 1955 diabetes mellitus was diagnosed. Tolbutamide therapy continued until 1964, then insulin therapy (depot insulin 36 units). Two weeks after the start of insulin therapy, erythema and induration developed at the injection site with pruritus and pricking sensations. Despite these symptoms, therapy was continued. There was no medical follow-up.

At the time of evaluation in hospital, a pale red, indurated area, 3 cm in diameter was seen at the injection site. This had been present for seven days. The symptoms were most intense 24 hours after the administration of insulin. Immunocytology showed by immunofluorescence 21%, by immune adherence 18%, especially marked among the granulocytes. The skin test showed delayed reaction to bovine and porcine insulin; the additive substances of the preparations used were negative. The serum evidenced markedly increased insulin-binding capacity: 160 units/liter for bovine insulin, 100 units/liter for porcine insulin. No skin-sensitizing antibodies against insulin were demonstrable. Insulin requirements were 68—76 units depot insulin (blood sugar 134 mg%, urine sugar 0.9 gm%). Therapy was continued since no transition to another insulin was possible.

Discussion. This patient manifested a delayed allergy against both bovine and porcine insulin, which began shortly after the initiation of insulin therapy in 1964, and after 2 years persisted in a milder form. At the same time serum antibodies against insulin had developed to an appreciable level. Cellular and humoral antibodies existed together. Due to the low degree of cutaneous reaction, the therapy was not altered.

Case History no. 4

I. Sch. 60-year-old female patient

In 1961 diabetes mellitus was diagnosed and treated with Rastinon. Due to high blood and urine sugar values (350 mg% and 3.0 gm% respectively), insulin therapy was begun on 24 Nov., 1965: mixed insulin (Depot-Hoechst) 32 units. Four days after the first injection, erythema and induration developed at the injection site with maximum intensity 12—18 hours after the injection of the insulin. At the evaluation in hospital on 2 Dec. 1965, a red induration 4 cm in diameter was seen on the upper right arm. Immunocytology showed by immunofluorescence 18% sensitized white cells, by immune adherence 18% (lymphocytes 9% and granulocytes 9%). Skin test was negative. Therapy continued with the same insulin preparation, and there was a spontaneous decline in the symptoms, with a decrease of 3 and 1% respectively in the number of sensitized cells. In the serum neither insulin-neutralizing nor skin-sensitizing antibodies were demonstrable.

Discussion. This patient manifested a short-lived state of delayed insulin allergy with the appearance of sensitized leukocytes. Under continuation of the therapy, desensitization occurred. There was no evidence of humoral antibodies.

Case History no. 5

Th. C. 68-year-old female patient

In 1962 diabetes mellitus was diagnosed and tolbutamide therapy was instituted. In January 1966 urine glucose excretion increased to 6 gm%, or 90 gm/24 hrs. and insulin therapy was started with combined insulin-depot insulin 32 units. Six days after the first injection, a painful erythema (4 cm in diameter) appeared at the injection site, maximum intensity being 20 hrs. after the insulin injection. With continuation of insulin therapy, the area of skin reaction increased to an induration of 7 cm in diameter both thighs. There was no essential effect on glucose metabolism (blood sugar 166 mg%, urine sugar 1 gm%). Immunocytology on 17 Feb. 1966 showed by immunofluorescence 25 %m, by immune adherence 22%; the lymphocytes and granulocytes were equally involved. There was no insulin-binding antibody in the serum and no reagins were demonstrable. For personal reasons, the patient left the hospital and returned three weaks later. Skin manifestations in the interval had almost completely disappeared, only small reactions persisting. The insulin-binding capacity of the serum was less than 5 units/liter for bovine and porcine insulin. Insulin requirement did not increase (blood sugar 142 mg%, urine sugar 0.8 mg%), and therapy was continued with mixed insulin (Depot-Hoechst) 36 units. After a further 6 weeks, there were no demonstrable antigen-binding white cells and no further skin manifestations.

Discussion. This patient manifested a short-lived delayed allergy to insulin, with the appearance of sensitized cells and subsequent desensitization during continued insulin therapy. Independently, however, a humoral antibody of the neutralizing type developed in small quantity. Skin-sensitizing antibodies (reagins) were not in evidence. No skin test was carried out.

Case History no. 6

L. Sch. 58-year-old female patient

In September 1958 diabetes mellitus was diagnosed. Diet was tried, then in 1960 sulfonylureas. Because of high urine glucose excretion, insulin therapy was started on 15 Feb. 1966: mixed insulin (Depot-Hoechst) 32 units. After three days mild symptoms of an allergic reaction were seen at the injection site, increasing on the subsequent days; intensity was greatest 12—18 hours after the injection. Glucose metabolism was not affected (blood sugar 180 mg%, urine sugarfree). On examination, a dark red induration (7 cm diameter), was seen on both thighs. Immunocytology showed by immunofluorescence (IF) 14%, by immune adherence (IA) 12%. The lymphocytes and granulocytes were equally involved. On 29 Feb. 1966 there was an increase in the skin reaction and an increase in the sensitized cells (IF 29%, IA 34%). On 4 March 1966 the leukocytes were separated by the glass pearl technique: 13% of lymphocytes and 57% of granulocytes indicated antigen-binding. With immune adherence, lymphocyte antigen-binding was 17%, while the granulocytes showed nearly complete immune cytolyses (see Fig. 13). Six days later repeated investigations showed a slight decline in the antigen-binding cells by immunofluorescence; immunocytolysis by incubation with complement and antigen unchanged. The skin test showed a moderately strong delayed reaction to bovine and porcine insulin, no reaction to Surfen and Chloreton. There were no demonstrable reagins in the serum and no increase in insulin-binding capacity. Within 8 days a gradual regression was seen in the skin manifestations and a decrease in the number of antigen-binding cells (by immunofluorescence, lymphocytes 12%, granulocytes 25%; by immune adherence: lymphocytes 13%, granulocytes 15%). Incubation of granulocytes with antigen and complement gave no indication of immune-cytolysis. A slight delayed local skin reaction persisted (diameter 3 cm).

At the peak of intensity of the skin reaction, an excisional skin biopsy was done. Findings were: lymphocytic infiltration in the region of the deep corium layers, especially perivascular; degenerative changes of the vessel walls, such as swelling and endothelial damage; lymphocytic infiltration of the areas of the skin appendages, sweat and sebaceous glands, with moderate edema; in the upper corium occasional vascular dilatation with moderate perivascular infiltration; cytological differentiation of the infiltrate showed it to be predominantly lymphocytes, also granulated eosinophils, and histocytes. This is representative of granulomatous hyperergic inflammation.

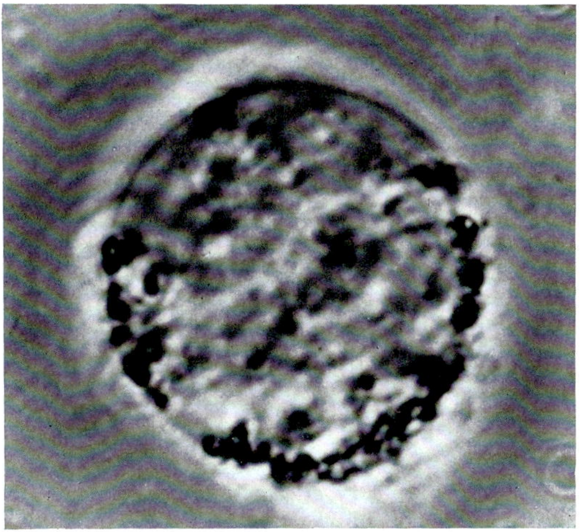

Fig. 13. Immune cytolysis of a granulocyte of a patient with long-lasting delayed allergy to insulin (incubation with antigen and complement). ×1600

Excision of another skin area into which insulin had been injected 48 hours before showed essentially mild infiltration of the vessels and skin appendages: dilated vessels, moderate edema of the mid-corium, slightly increased lymphocytic infiltration in the region of the upper corium. Cytological differentiation showed essentially only lymphocytic elements.

Immune histology: after incubation of several cryostat sections of the skin biopsy specimen with an FITC-labelled guinea pig anti-bovine insulin serum (globulin fraction), there was no specific uptake by cells or tissue structures (Fig. 14 a); incubation of several cryostat sections with FITC-labelled bovine insulin showed uptake by some mononuclear cells lying perivascularly (Fig. 14 b). Controls with FITC-labelled bovine serum albumin (BSA) as well as pure FITC evidenced no uptake. Incubation of the tissue with unlabelled insulin as pretreatment had as a result a marked suppression of specific uptake.

Discussion. This patient manifested a delayed allergic reaction to bovine and porcine insulin which reached its maximum 2 to 3 weeks after the onset of insulin therapy. The symptoms declined in intensity, but were not

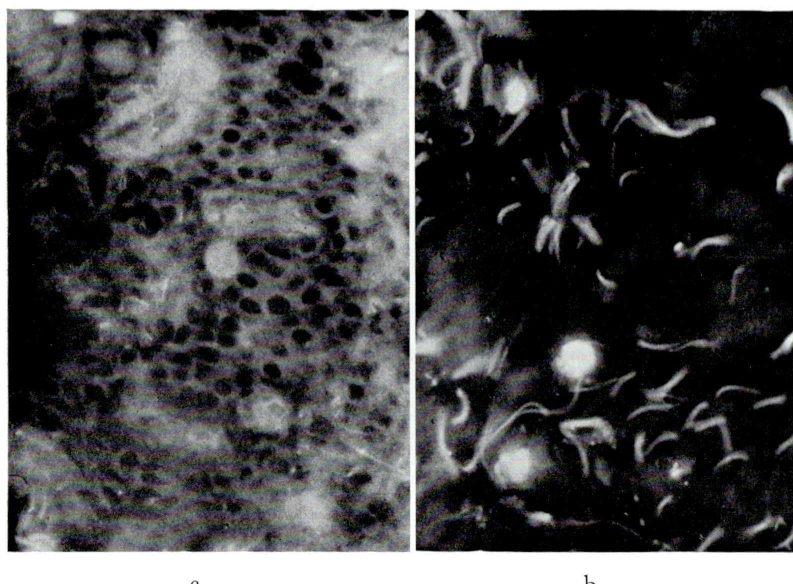

a b

Fig. 14. Immunohistological evaluation of a skin biopsy of a patient with delayed insulin allergy. a Incubation with FITC-labelled antibody to insulin (no fluorescence); b Incubation with FITC-labelled insulin. (Binding of antigen by 3 cells of the infiltrate). Cryostat section. ×480

yet fully resolved. The delayed immune reaction predominated, but was accompanied by antigen-reactions of humoral antibodies. The swelling of the vessel walls indicated that this was not just a pure delayed reaction. Humoral antibodies must have participated, even if not demonstrable with the present methods. This probably represents a combined type in the sense of a markedly "delayed" immediate response.

Case History no. 7

J. Sch., 54-year-old female patient

In 1963 diabetes mellitus was diagnosed and treated with sulfonylureas. Because of elevated urine sugar excretion, insulin therapy (mixed bovine-porcine insulin (Depot-Hoechst) 32 units) was started on 31 March 1966. A few days after the initiation of insulin therapy (the patient's account is not precise), an erythema measuring 8 cm in diameter developed at the injection site, with a maximum intensity after 14 hours. Evaluation in the hospital three weeks later showed moderately large induration (3 cm diameter) on both thighs and a weaker induration in the areas injected during the last 7 days. Immune cytology: Immunofluorescence 12%; immune adherence 11%; lymphocytes and granulocytes equally involved. The skin test showed weak reaction of the delayed type against bovine and porcine insulin; a repeat evaluation on 5 May indicated clear regression of the skin manifestations; only 5% and 6% antigen-binding cells, respectively. In the serum the maximum insulin-binding capacity was 0.5 units/liter for bovine and porcine insulin. There were no demonstrable reagins in the serum. A further repeat evaluation on 2 June showed no skin manifestations; no sensitized cells in blood.

Discussion. This patient represents a predominantly delayed insulin allergy to bovine and porcine insulin. Spontaneous desensitization occurred under continued therapy with regression of all manifestations. As far as could be demonstrated, there was no concurrent humoral antibody formation.

Case History no. 8

M. W., 67-year-old female patient

In 1958 diabetes mellitus was diagnosed and treated with tolbutamide. In 1964 insulin therapy was begun in an out-lying hospital as glucose metabolism was inadequate. The therapy induced an intense localized allergic manifestation and had to be discontinued. Treatment continued with sulfonylureas. On 7 February 1966, blood sugar was 232% and urine sugar 6.6% = 110 gm/24 hours. Another attempt was made to employ insulin therapy (mixed insulin (Depot-Hoechst) 32 units). 4 days later a dark red induration (3 cm diameter) was seen 12—24 hours after an injection (see Fig. 15). The induration progressed rapidly during the next few days, causing intense pain, and the patient was admitted to hospital. A skin test showed delayed reaction to bovine insulin, no reaction to porcine insulin or the additive substances. On 21 March immune cytology showed immunofluorescence 18%, immune adherence 15%; respective involvement: in the immunofluorescence 13% lymphocytes and 16% granulocytes; in the immune adherence 10% lymphocytes and 8% granulocytes. 12 days later a localized immediate reaction (Fig. 16) occurred at the injection site, followed by a severe generalized urticaria (Fig. 17) after the next insulin injection one day later with Quincke edema, glottal edema and hypotension (a generalized immediate reaction to insulin). Therapy was begun with cortisone, calcium and antihistamines. Continuing this therapy, it was possible to give pure porcine insulin without any allergic manifestations. Antigen-binding cells in blood regressed to normal values; the insulin-binding capacity of the serum during the generalized urticaria was 35 units/liter to bovine insulin and 2 units/liter to porcine insulin. In the allergic serum transfer test in rhesus monkeys, positive evidence of reagins was obtained (Fig. 18). There was thus clear evidence of a thermo-labile skin-sensitizing antibody to insulin.

Discussion. As a consequence of sensitization to insulin 2 years before, the patient, after approximately 4 weeks of persistent delayed allergy and simultaneous formation of humoral antibodies of the neutralizing type,

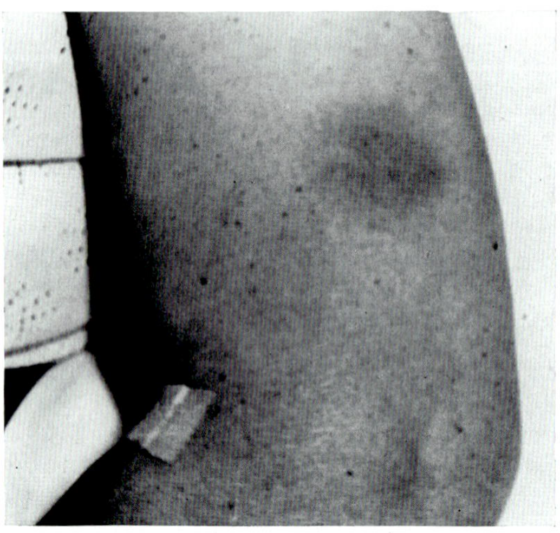

Fig. 15. Mild delayed allergic reaction to insulin 24 hours after the injection on day 4 of treatment (case no. 8)

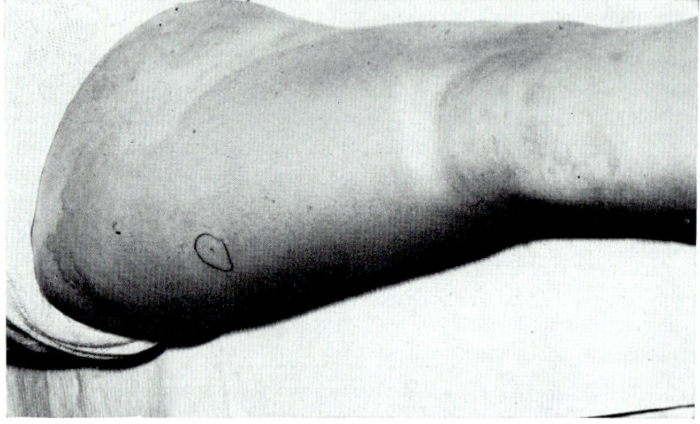

Fig. 16. Local immediate allergic reaction to insulin 30 min after the injection (case no. 8)

abruptly developed skin-sensitizing antibodies, i. e. a "turn-about" of delayed, local allergy into a generalized allergy of the immediate type. Sensitized cells and humoral antibodies were directly exclusively against bovine insulin (Fig. 19).

Case History no. 9

J. Sch., 65-year-old female patient

In 1961 diabetes mellitus was diagnosed and treated with sulfonylureas, changed after a few weeks to insulin. Insulin requirements were so

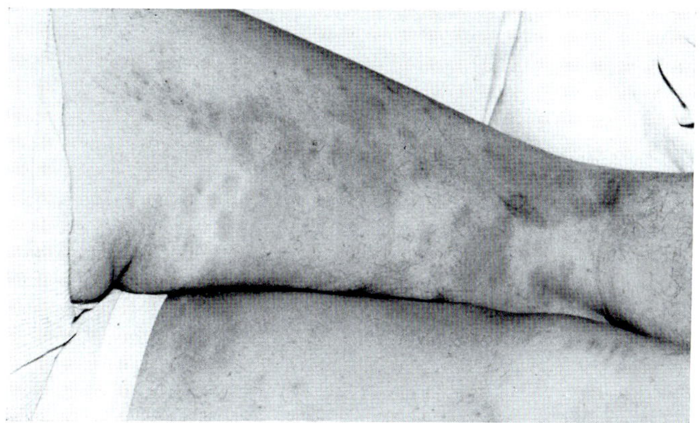

Fig. 17. Generalized urticaria in the same case

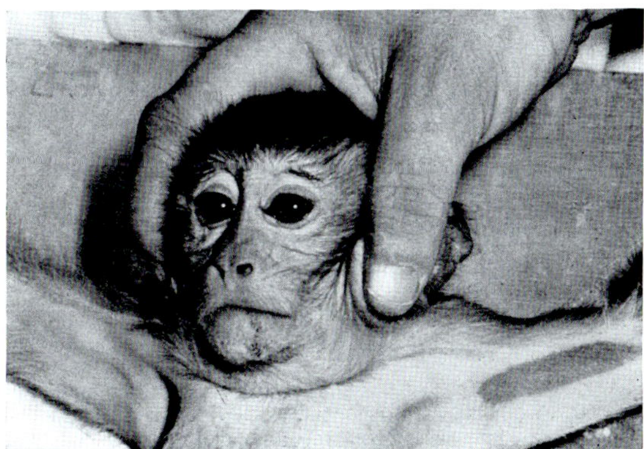

Fig. 18. Demonstration of reagins in serum of case no. 8 with the allergic serum transfer test according to LAYTON et al. (1965). Rhesus monkey. Left arm: Extravasation of the dye (injected with antigen) at the place where patient's serum was injected intradermally 48 hours before. Right arm: negative reaction with heat-inactivated serum of the patient

low that treatment reverted to sulfonylureas until 1965. On 25 November, 1965, insulin therapy was again started (mixed bovine-porcine insulin (Depot) 36 units). 8 days later, for the first time, a painful erythema occurred at the injection sites, approximately palm-sized in diameter, and reaching maximum intensity after 16 hours. Blood sugar was 194 mg%; urine sugar 2.4 gm%. On 13 December, approximately one hour after insulin injection,

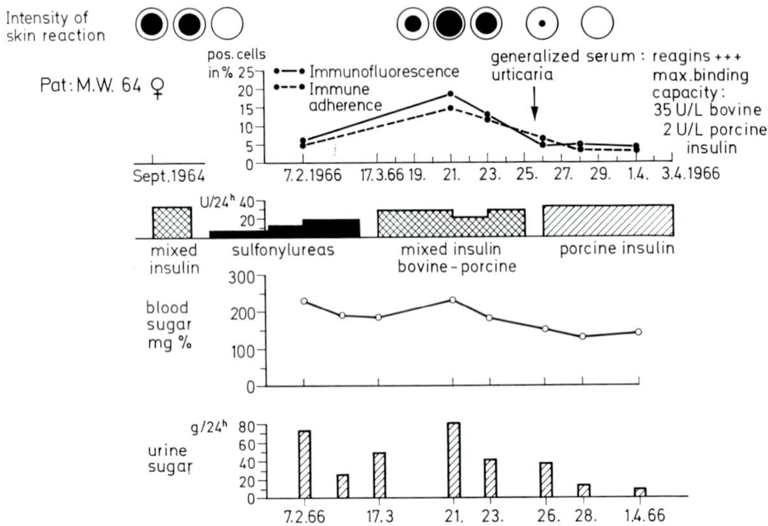

Fig. 19. Diagram of the course of case no. 8. Increasing number of insulin-binding white blood cells paralleling the intensity of the skin reaction. Decrease after switching from delayed to immediate form of insulin allergy

a generalized urticaria developed, with Quinke edema and glottal edema (of low intensity). Treatment with Neobridal caused regression of symptoms. Despite continuation of insulin therapy, there were no further signs of an immediate allergy, but the local delayed allergy as before. Immunocytology on 17 December showed immunofluorescence 15%, immune adherence 14%, and on 20 December immunofluorescence 18%, immune adherence 18%. Granulocytes were the predominant reactive cells. Maximum insulin-binding capacity was less than 0.5 unit/liter; skin test negative. With continued insulin therapy, there was regression of these manifestations and the antigen-binding cells fell to 3% (immunofluorescence) and to 1% (immune adherence).

Discussion. After sensitization to insulin 4 years previously delayed insulin allergy appeared and persisted for three weeks with a brief appearance of skin-sensitizing antibodies, which were very probably directed against insulin, although no reliable evidence could be obtained (additional antigens were not demonstrable). With continued insulin therapy, the skin allergy spontaneously disappeared (desensitization).

Case History no. 10

J. H., 43-year-old female patient

In 1961 diabetes mellitus was diagnosed and treated with Rastinon; after a few weeks this was changed to insulin, but discontinued due to allergic skin reactions, sulfonylurea therapy being reinstituted. In 1962 metabolic deterioration necessitated renewal of insulin therapy. Local delayed skin allergy again occurred, but the same insulin preparation (mixed bovine-porcine insulin (Depot-Hoechst)) was continued in increase doses. Immunocytology showed immunofluorescence 21%, immune adherence 20% and 28%. Granulocytes were the predominating antigen-binding cells. Intramuscular injection caused regression of the cell percentage and the skin manifestations. Renewed manifestations were seen when the subcutaneous injection technique was resumed. Prolonged incubation of leukocytes with antigen and complement led to complete immune cytolysis; there were no humoral antibodies of either the neutralizing or reagin type.

Discussion. This patient represents a state of delayed hypersensitivity to bovine and porcine insulin existing for one year. The sensitized cells, in contrast to the antigen, were more sensitive to the technique of immune adherence (with the presence of complement) than to the technique of immunofluorescence. The repeatedly observed appearance of immunecytolysis could represent the existence of a highly-active cellular antibody whose concentration in the serum is too low to be demonstrable by the given methods.

Case History no. 11

K. W., 62-year-old male patient

In 1964 diabetes mellitus was diagnosed and treated with sulfonylureas. On 1 August 1966, treatment was changed to insulin because of co-existing chronic liver disease, despite adequate control previously.

On 4 August 1966, the first manifestation of a dark red infiltration was seen at the injection sites, progressing in the subsequent days to palm-sized, with maximum intensity 18—24 hours after injection. On 12 August, due to progression of the allergy, sulfonylurea therapy was reinstituted. After 8 days, for reasons which are not clear insulin therapy was restarted. On admission to hospital a 5 cm diameter, indurated skin infiltration of the previous injection sites was observed. Skin tests showed a clear delayed reaction to bovine insulin and a weak reaction to porcine; the reaction against additives of the insulin charge was negative. Immunocytology showed immunofluorescence 7%; immune adherence 8%, and 4 days later immunofluorescence 12%; immune adherence 10%. Under continued insulin therapy, there was regression of the skin lesions and a decline of the antigen-binding cells to normal values. Control evaluation on 9 September 1966 showed no skin reaction.

Discussion. This patient presents a 2-week (approximately) existing delayed allergy to bovine insulin (less to porcine), which spontaneously regressed under further insulin therapy.

Case History no. 12

G. R., 66-year-old female patient

In 1955 diabetes mellitus was diagnosed and treated by diet control until 1961; sulfonylurea therapy since 1961.

On 22 February, 1966, insulin therapy was started due to elevated urine sugar excretion (5.4 gm⁰/₀). After 4 days a delayed allergic reaction produced a bright red lesion, 3—4 cm in diameter. With continued therapy

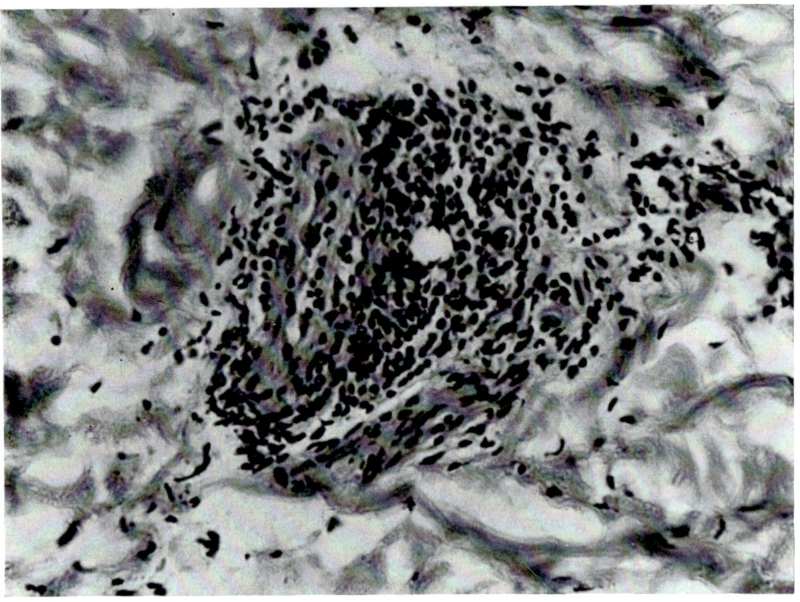

Fig. 20. Skin biopsy of case no. 12. Perivascular infiltration with mononuclear cells. Tuberculin type reaction. Giemsa staining. ×180

there was no alteration in the infiltrate, whose maximum intensity was 18 hours after the injection. Immunocytology showed immunofluorescence 9%, immune adherence 8%. On 17 March, immunofluorescence 28%, immune adherence 32%. Cell type: predominantly lymphocytes. A skin biopsy was done: histological evaluation showed edema of the upper corium, in part a massive perivascular infiltration by round cells and striking degranulation of the perivascular mast cells, approximately half evidencing degranulation. The predominant cells were from the lymphocyte series, granulocytes remaining in the background, the general state representative of a delayed reaction similar to the tuberculin type (Fig. 20). Immunohistology: after incubation with an FITC-labelled antibovine insulin serum (globulin-fraction), there was no special uptake by cells or vessel walls, but after incubation with FITC-labelled bovine insulin, there was uptake by single cells in the inflammatory infiltrate.

Maximum insulin-binding capacity of the serum was less than 0.5 units/liter (normal value); no demonstrable reagins. Under continued insulin therapy a spontaneous regression of the skin lesions occurred and the antigen-binding cells returned to normal values.

Discussion. This patient presents a state of delayed allergy to insulin of short duration. Histologically the typical findings of delayed reaction were seen. Spontaneous remission (desensitization) occurred under continued insulin therapy.

Case History no. 13

J. B., 50-year-old female patient

Diabetes mellitus was detected in 1963 and treated initially with sulfonylureas; since November 1965, insulin. Five days after the first insulin injection, a painful erythema and induration appeared at the injection site, showing maximum intensity after 14 hours. In the following days, the infiltrated area progressed to a diameter of 7 cm; there was then a slow regression to 1—2 cm diameter. Therapy was continued and, after another 6 months, recurrent minimal skin reactions led to evaluation and admission to hospital. On 6 June 1966 immunocytology showed immunofluorescence 7%, immune adherence 8%; no further differentiation was possible. The skin test clearly showed a delayed reaction to bovine and porcine insulin. In the serum the maximum binding capacity for both bovine and porcine insulin was 50 units/liter. There were no demonstrable reagins. Blood sugar was 200 gm%; urine sugar 1.5 gm%. Therapy continued with depot insulin 32 units. No further evaluation was possible, since the patient no longer appeared for consultation.

Discussion. This was a case of delayed allergy to bovine and porcine insulin with severe reactions during the initial insulin therapy, but with only a weak residuum over a 7 months period. There was simultaneous development of humoral antibodies of the neutralizing type.

Case History no. 14

H. H., 44-year-old female patient

In 1963 diabetes mellitus was diagnosed and treated with sulfonylureas.

In March 1966 insulin therapy was started because of high blood and urine sugar values. After a few days a local, delayed skin reaction appeared which was not affected by changing the insulin preparations. After several weeks sulfonylurea treatment was reinstituted but gave no satisfactory control of the diabetes (fasting blood sugar 196 mg%, urine sugar 8 gm%). Insulin therapy was again attempted: on the second day, 12 hours after injection, erythema measuring 2 cm in diameter appeared with induration and itching and pricking sensations, which were especially severe at night, i. e. 16 to 20 hours after the injection. Symptoms increased in intensity in the following days. The skin test showed clearly a delayed reaction to bovine insulin, weak reaction to porcine insulin, no reaction to additive substances. Immunocytology on 29 August 1966: immunofluorescence 19%, immune adherence negative due to technical error; on 2 September: immunofluorescence 15%, immune adherence 16%; on 5 September: immunofluorescence 14%, immune adherence 15%; on 7 September: immunofluorescence 16%, immune adherence 15%; on 9 September: immunofluorescence 14%, immune adherence 17%. The majority of the cells binding FITC-insulin at this time were mononuclear, i. e. lymphoid types. Under continued insulin therapy, the skin reaction appeared sooner (after 8 hours), but was less intense. Immunocytology on 15 September: immunofluorescence 18%, immune adherence 16%; on 16 September: immunofluorescence 11%, immune adherence 12%; on 23 September: immunofluorescence 9%, immune adherence 8%. Cell types were predominantly granulocytes.

Serum antibody investigations on 29 August showed maximum insulin-binding capacity of 30 units/liter; on 16 September: 180 units/liter; on 23 September: 42 units/liter (results for porcine insulin). The patient refused further investigations.

Discussion. This patient presents a quite acute development of delayed insulin allergy, after insulin therapy had been begun but terminated six months previously. Continued therapy led to a regression of the symptoms, without full disappearance. During the period of delayed allergy neutralizing antibodies were demonstrable. The reinstitution of insulin therapy after earlier discontinuation due to allergy, must be seen as a boosting effect.

Addendum. In 3 cases (female patients), not described in detail, there was a delayed allergic reaction to insulin at the beginning of treatment but no significant binding of insulin by peripheral blood cells could be observed. In all these patients only one examination of blood cells was performed. The reason for the negative results remained unclear. Repeated investigations were not possible for various reasons. In two of the patients a skin test was performed but evidenced no skin reactivity to insulin or the additives.

b) Summary of the Findings

α) Clinical Picture

The skin manifestations of the patients previously evaluated had the following pattern: at the earliest 6 hours, usually 10—12 hours but occasionally as much as 24 hours after the administration of insulin, there developed at the site of injection a colorless or dull-red induration, accompanied by burning sensations and troublesome itching. These events reached maximum intensity usually after approximately 24 hours, rarely earlier, and occasionally later. The traces of this inflammatory reaction were generally apparent to sight and touch even 2—3 days afterwards, sometimes as long as one week after the injection. In some patients, a bright red unclearly demarcated area developed in the center of the dusky erythema. The extent of the skin reaction varied from 3 to 10 cm in diameter. The reactions occurring at injection sites on the thigh were generally larger than those at sites on the arm. However, subjectively allergic reactions on the arm were found more distressing than those in the leg. In 4 of the patients the skin manifestations first occurred 4—5 days after the first insulin injection. In another 4 diabetics the initial allergic reactions began months, and in one case even 2 years, previously, so that no exact report of the first appearance could be ascertained. Another six patients had already been treated with insulin much earlier, and the therapy had had to be discontinued because of allergy. The reinstitution of therapy saw the occurrence of cutaneous allergy on the 2nd or 3rd day after the first injection, therefore earlier than in those diabetics who were receiving insulin for the first time.

β) Antigen-binding by Sensitized White Blood Cells

By means of immunofluorescence and immune adherence tests, binding of insulin to the surface of circulating blood cells could be demonstrated in all patients who were evaluated with three exceptions (see page 68). The number of reacting cells generally paralleled the intensity of the skin reactions, as is particularly well shown in Case no. 1 where a replacement of bovine insulin by porcine insulin resulted in a regression of the skin reaction as well as a marked decrease of the sensitized cells. Only in 4 cases did the number of reactive blood cells seem higher than would be expected in view of the weak cutaneous reactions. This occurred especially in fading reactions, so that apparently the reaction of the blood cells lasted longer than the cutaneous inflammatory process. The opposite was never observed, i. e. that a strong cutaneous reaction should ensue without an elevation of sensitized blood cells. Equal value was attached to both cytological methods employed, as shown in Fig. 21. The number of antigen-binding cells in non-diabetics and in insulin-treated diabetics without allergic cutaneous manifestations was at most 6%, and usually lay between 1 and 3%.

When one evaluated preparations of mixed white blood cells by means of immunofluorescence, single lymphocytes as well as granulocytes were seen to be bound to the labelled insulin (Figs. 10 and 11). An adequate spreading of the cytoplasm so as to display the nuclei upon the siliconized surface of the glass slide is necessary for the differentiation of the cells. Attempts to restain the preparation with Pappenheim's panoptic stain yielded unsatisfactory results. In some patients the white blood cells were fractionated in a glass-bead column before incubation with FITC insulin. In instances of good separation, the lymphocytes were occasionally "contaminated" with 5—10% granulocytes (as examined by panoptic staining). In contrast, the granulocytes were nearly "pure". Counts of cells which had bound labelled insulin, showed that the values were not absolute, but only relative. This was especially true of the lymphocytes. They do not adhere very readily to a glass surface, so that a large number of the cells are always lost during the incubation with antigen or during the

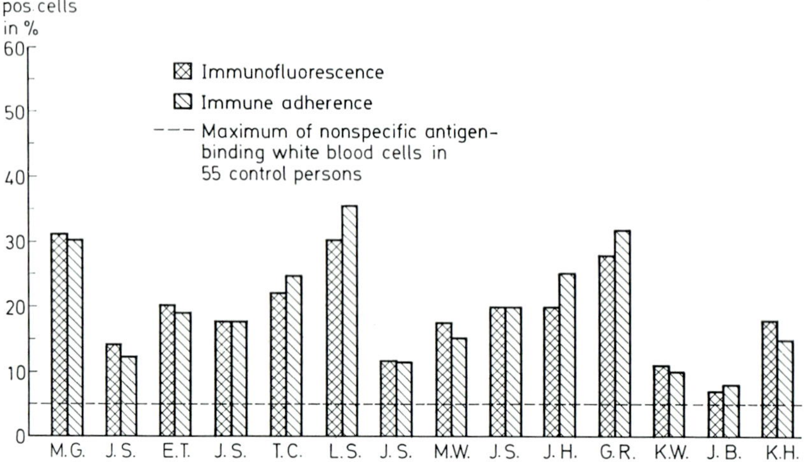

Fig. 21. Number of antigen-binding cells from the peripheral blood evaluated with immunofluorescence and immune adherence (not absolute numbers for technical reasons, see discussion) in patients with delayed insulin allergy

subsequent washings. Since occasionally a surprisingly large percentage of fixed lymphocytes showed specific insulin binding, it could be that the sensitized cells — in the presence of antigen — have an increased adhesiveness. For this hypothesis there is also support. PLOTZ and TALLAL (1967) found that splenic antibody-forming cells had a greater stickiness to glass surfaces than normal spleen cells. In general the investigations with immune adherence supported these

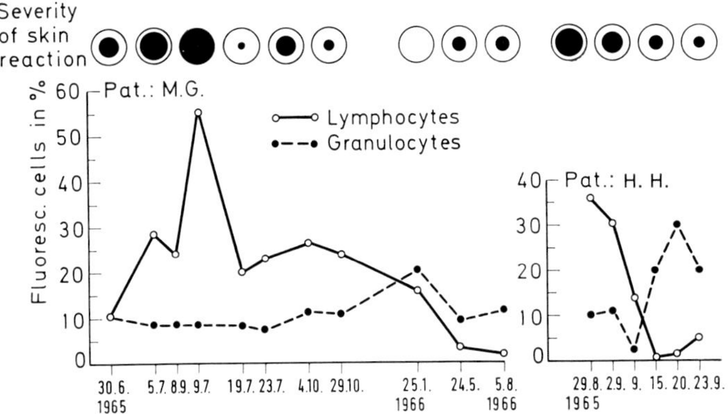

Fig. 22. Behaviour of antigen-binding white blood cells in two patients with delayed insulin allergy. Correlation between severity of the skin reaction and number of antigen-binding lymphocytes. No correlation between skin reaction and antigen binding by granulocytes

assumptions. The number of reacting lymphocytes was less than in immunofluorescence.

The granulocytes gave a better correspondence between the number of antigen-binding cells measured with both techniques. Granulocytes adhere more readily to a siliconized surface, so that fewer cells are lost during antigen binding and washing.

In 2 patients it was possible to make frequent evaluations of blood cells by immunofluorescence from the beginning of the insulin allergy, and to obtain data over a long period. It became clear that more lymphocytes reacted initially with the antigen, granulocytes reacting later (Fig. 22). In patients whose initial stage of insulin allergy had already passed at the time of evaluation, virtually only the granulocytes reacted in vitro with the antigen.

It seems appropriate to make the eosinophils responsible for the reaction between granulocytes and antigen in immunofluorescence. These cells have repeatedly been found to possess an unspecific affinity for fluorescein-isothiocyanate (see literature in NAIRN, 1964). However, in the patients studied, the number of eosinophils paralleled the number of antigen-binding cells in only one case (Fig. 23). In all other patients there was no correlation.

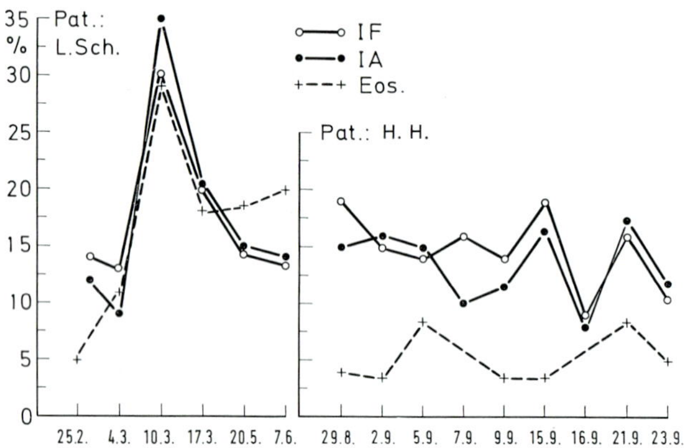

Fig. 23. Number of eosinophils and antigen-binding white blood cells. Among all patients with delayed insulin allergy only one showed a parallel increase and decrease, suggesting that antigen-binding cells consisted of eosinophils (left side). In all other patients no correlation was observed as in case no. 14 (right side)

The sensitized cells, in respect to antigen binding, present the following picture:

a) Immunofluorescence: lymphocytes and granulocytes have an equally homogeneous or granular staining of the cytoplasm. The nucleus (and nuclear segments) stand out distinctly as darkened areas, and contain no fluorescing structure. In comparison to normal blood cell preparations, the cytoplasm was essentially more spread out as a consequence of the siliconized surface.

b) Immune adherence: sensitized cells demonstrated a binding of 1, 2, 3 or more erythrocytes on their surface, occasionally a complete occupation of the leukocyte surface by a wreath of erythrocytes could be found (the rosette phenomenon, see Fig. 12). In three cases the incubation of the sensitized cells with antigen and complement induces immune-cytolysis, the beginning stage of which is seen in Fig. 13.

The sensitized cells manifested antigen binding not only for bovine but also for porcine insulin, in both immunofluorescence and in immune adherence. This was also observed in those cases where the allergy was directed predominantly against bovine insulin. The non-homogeneity of therapeutic insulin preparations (in general, the insulin mixture used by the patients at that time contained 70% bovine insulin and 30% or less porcine insulin) did not permit an answer to the question: do the sensitized cells have a greater specificity in vivo than in vitro?

Investigations for specificity. The immune adherence technique is in effect an in vitro method which indicates sensitized cells without use of a dye, and may be used in parallel with immunofluorescence investigations. The specificity of the results of immunofluorescence are thus satisfactorily controlled. As shown in Fig. 21, antigen binding of sensitized cells was found with both methods in nearly equal numbers. — The essential controls for the immunofluorescence method were done by preincubation with unlabelled insulin (inhibition technique), with FITC-bovine serum albumin and with free dye. Furthermore, cells of normal persons were examined with FITC-insulin. It was shown that the inhibition technique gave, not complete, but marked suppression of the specific fluorescence. With labelled BSA and free dye, no substantial unspecific staining of the cells occurred. Cells of normal persons were stained by FITC-insulin unspecifically up to 6% (mainly 1—3%). — In some cases the sandwich technique was tried, i. e. incubation of the sensitized cells with unlabelled insulin and afterwards with FITC-labelled insulin antibody. But this technique always gave disappointing results, because a weak fluorescence was observed in nearly all cells. Interestingly, PARKER, ELEVITCH and GRODSKY (1963) were also unable to detect antibody-producing cells against insulin with this method. They found, as in the present study, that direct immunofluorescence, i. e. incubation with labelled antigen, was the only reliable fluorescent method.

Because eosinophilic cells are known to possess a tendency to unspecific uptake of fluorochromes, patients were examined who had eosinophilic cells of other etiologies (penicillin allergy, ascaridiasis, reticulosis). While in a few cases the eosinophils showed a certain affinity for all FITC-labelled proteins, this was not so in other patients. Thus no empirical rule could be defined and unspecific fluorescence as an consequence of staining of eosinophils is excluded as a cause of binding of FITC-insulin by granulocytes.

The significance of species specificity in the antigenicity of insulin was shown in 3 out of 14 patients with delayed allergic reaction. The allergy was directed toward bovine insulin; the skin reaction and the number of sensitized cells regressed after this was replaced by pure porcine insulin.

γ) Behaviour of Serum Antibodies

According to the investigations of various authors (for literature see Berson and Yalow, 1959 b), neutralizing antibodies develop after a greater or lesser period of time in all diabetics treated with insulin. Our investigations raise the intriguing question whether the humoral antibodies are already present at the time of onset of the sensitized cells. The maximum insulin-binding capacity was employed as the criterion for the existence and level of humoral anti-insulin antibodies, simultaneously with the passive hemagglutination test on the serum according to Arquilla and Stavitsky (1956 a). The relationship to the cellular antibodies is shown in Table 3, page 75. It can be seen that, in those patients who received insulin for the first time and developed a delayed allergy shortly thereafter, there was a period, however short, during which sensitized cells were present. The techniques used were not able to demonstrate humoral antibodies. Then, after varying lengths of time, the circulating antibodies appeared; thus, in Case no. 1, after 10 days. On the other hand, Case 10, even 2 years after the onset of continuing skin reactions, still showed no definite proof of humoral antibodies. In 2 other cases who had already received insulin at an earlier time, there existed even at the time of the first injection (Case 8: 7 days; Case 14: 2 days) after the renewal of insulin therapy, a high binding capacity for insulin which indicated the existence of humoral neutralizing anti-insulin antibodies. During the stage of delayed anti-insulin allergy, the serum of the patients being investigated contained no reagins, as was demonstrable in monkeys using the AST test (allergic serum transfer test) according to Layton et al. (1965).

Table 3. *Synopsis of duration of the delayed allergy to insulin in 14 patients, existence of antigen binding cells in blood and humoral insulin antibodies examined by different methods*

Case No.	Pat.	Duration of Allergy	Sensitized Cells	Max. IBC [a] U/L	Titer with passive Haemaggl.	Reagins
14	H. H.	2 days (6 months before: Insulin)	+	15	30	ϕ
		11 days	+	60	90	ϕ
8	M. W.	3 days	+	?	ϕ	ϕ
		1964 short period of insulin therapy (7th day: immediate type allergy)	ϕ	35	ϕ	+
1	M. G.	3 days	+	<0.5	ϕ	ϕ
		10 days	+	60	30	ϕ
4	I. S.	5 days	+	<0.5	ϕ	ϕ
12	G. R.	13 days	+	<0.5	ϕ	ϕ
11	K. W.	14 days	+	<0.5	10	ϕ
6	L. S.	3 weeks	+	<0.5	ϕ	ϕ
7	J. S.	3 weeks	+	<0.5	ϕ	ϕ
9	I. S.	3 weeks	+	<0.5	ϕ	ϕ
2	I. S.	4 weeks	+	40	ϕ	ϕ
5	T. C.	5 weeks	+	5	ϕ	ϕ
13	I. B.	8 months	+	50	30	ϕ
3	E. T.	20 months	+	160	ϕ	ϕ
10	I. H.	2 years	+	<0.5	ϕ	ϕ
15	W. V.	— (5 years immediate type allergy)	ϕ	<0.5	ϕ	+

[a] Insulin-Binding Capacity.

The investigation was positive, however, in a male patient with immediate allergy to insulin which had existed for 15 years (Case 15, W. V.) and in a female patient (Case 8, M. W.) whose brief status of delayed insulin allergy suddenly blossomed into an immediate allergy with generalized urticaria (Fig. 17, page 63).

δ) *Cytophilic Antibodies*

The incubation of leukocytes of healthy controls with the serum of patients who demonstrated a delayed skin allergy and numerous sensitized blood cells was negative. There was no evidence of the existence of the so-called cytophilic antibody, which had been found to be the cause of the reactivity of sensitized cells with antibody in various animal species (Boyden and Sorkin, 1961; Sorkin, 1963; Boyden, 1963, 1964).

Our own results, based on immunofluorescence, yielded consistently negative results, i. e. the percentage of fluorescing cells (present to a small extent even in normal subjects) did not increase after the addition of serum from our allergic diabetics.

ε) *Histological Findings of Skin Biopsies*

In three out of the fourteen patients evaluated, it was possible to investigate the affected skin areas histologically; the variable results reflect the various possibilities. They suggest an isolated occurrence of sensitized cells with a simultaneous distribution of humoral antibodies. Thus, in Case 12, the cutaneous biopsy 14 days after the onset of allergy manifested a characteristic isolated delayed reaction (Fig. 20). A massive perivascular round-cell infiltration and a significant degranulation of the mast cells were found. The granulocytes remained entirely in the background. The biopsy of Case 6 demonstrated a granulomatous hyperergic inflammation. There was a perivascular lymphocytic infiltration with accompanying eosinophilia and histiocytic components, and also a swelling of individual vessel walls with endothelial damage. This instance suggests humoral antibody involvement, although the maximum insulin-binding capacity was not high (0.5 units/liter). Another cutaneous site of the same patient demonstrated minimal infiltration of the vessels with significant edema of the mid-corium and only a mild lymphocytic infiltration of the upper corium: this picture is more in keeping with a simple delayed reaction. Even more removed from the pure delayed reaction, i. e. approaching nearer to the early anaphylactic reaction, were the alterations present in Case 1. An edematous saturation and swelling of the vessel walls occurred, as well as a moderate perivascular round-cell infiltration, with granulocytes and single eosinophils, which appeared to be attached to the subepidermal blisters. These changes were designated as an anaphylactic reaction of the immediate type with transition to the hyperergic granulomatous reaction. The single delayed reaction stage had already occurred 7 months before in this case. The patient manifested, as previously, a delayed allergy to insulin although a clearly elevated maximal insulin-binding capacity (i. e. humoral antibodies) had in the meanwhile developed.

These three cases had in common that they represented clinically a delayed skin reaction and antigen binding with their circulating leukocytes. They differed, however, in the humoral antibody distribution reflected in the localized cutaneous inflammatory involvement and in the intensity — in part weaker, in part stronger — of the manifestations of early and delayed reactions to the same antigen.

Immunohistological investigation of cryostat sections of the same excised tissue failed to demonstrate that the antigen utilized an FITC-labelled anti-insulin antibody (not even demonstrable in the swollen vessel walls). Individual cells of the inflammatory infiltrate did stand out, however, with the labelled insulin fluorescence (Fig. 14, page 60).

ζ) Findings with Lymphocyte Transformation

In six diabetics with an insulin allergy, the transformation ability of blood lymphocytes to blast forms was investigated by the in vitro addition of antigen. As had been shown in 1968 (FEDERLIN, KRIEGBAUM and FLAD), this phenomenon of blast transformation was demonstrable not only in two cases of generalized urticaria (immediate allergy) but in 4 patients with a localized delayed allergic reaction as (Fig. 24 a—c, Table 4). The technique consisted of the addition of 50 μg of bovine insulin per ml of incubation mixture, resulting in a marked increase in the number of transformed cells as compared with lymphocytes cultivated for 5 days without antigen. The standard was the transformation rate with phytohemagglutinin. An increase of the antigen dose to 500 μg/ml (10 fold) led to no further stimulation. Insulin-treated diabetics (5) without allergic manifestations responded with just as little lymphocyte transformation after insulin incubation as non-diabetics.

7. Discussion

From these investigations it is apparent that the frequently observed clinical signs of localized delayed allergy during insulin therapy by no means reflect incompatibility to some accompanying substances. Indeed, this appears to be a delayed immune reaction to the insulin antigen itself. Allergic reactions to disinfecting or stabilizing substances, such as are found in various insulin preparations, do occur, but quite seldom. Insulin is certainly not to be considered a weak antigen, as was maintained even a few years ago. The investi-

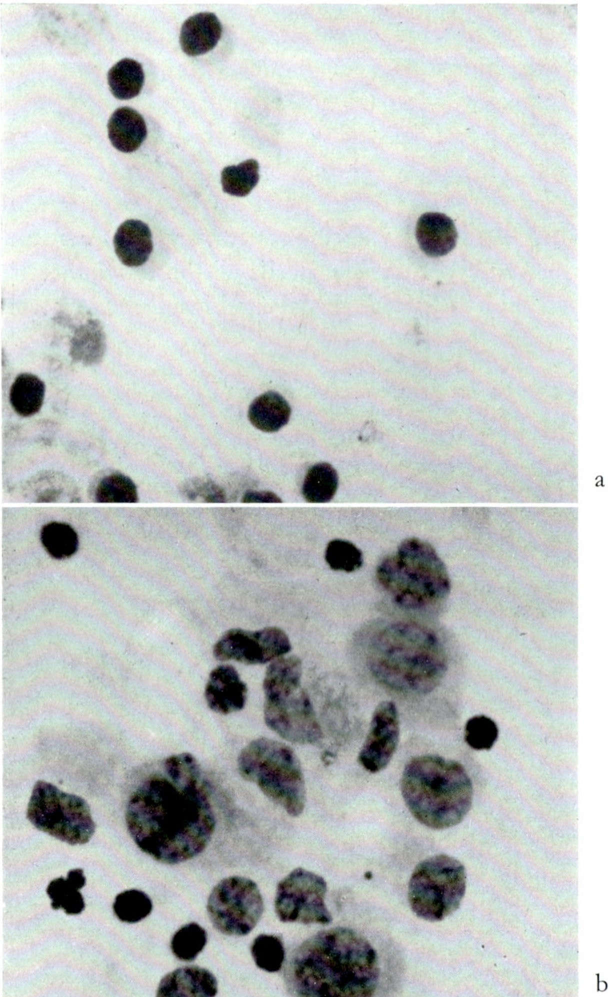

Fig. 24 a—b. Lymphocyte culture of a patient with immediate-type allergy to insulin: a After 5 days cultivation in normal tissue culture medium; b After 3 days with PHA

gations of SELA (1966) produced synthetic polypeptides with essentially smaller molecules which served as good immunogens. The high content of aromatic amino acid in insulin and its rigid molecular structure tend to strengthen its immunogenicity, which is further enhanced by the fact that the hormone is injected subcutaneously and

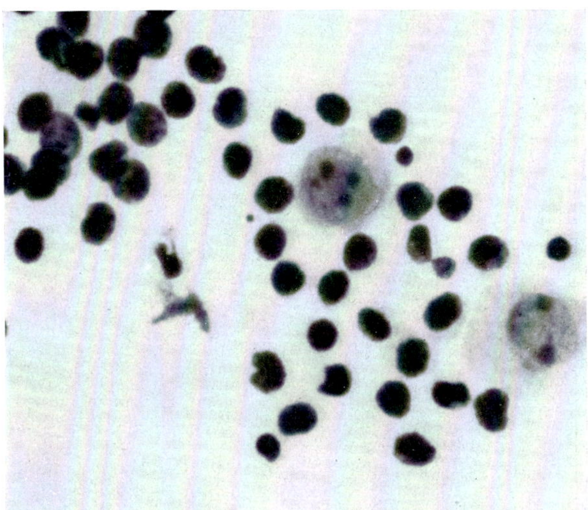

Fig. 24 c. After 5 days with antigen (insulin). Note blast transformation by antigen in c according to the PHA-induced stimulation of lymphocytes in b. Pappenheim staining. ×420

frequently given in depot form (crystallized or combined with a carrier). The prolonged and steady resorption is an additional reason for the development of immune reactions, in this case for the development of delayed-type allergy, as well as for later antibody formation.

These investigations also helped in the classification of purely external manifestations of allergic reactions of the delayed type by additional in vitro procedures, skin tests, and histologic examination of the skin. It was concluded that delayed allergic reactions were indeed possible as a temporary state in practically every diabetic. The number of patients who gave a history of allergic reaction truly appeared to depend upon the closeness of the clinical supervision. The files of the Diabetic Service of the Frankfurt University Clinic show that in 1964 only 3 patients out of 65 and in 1965 3 out of 77 reported such symptoms to the physician; but in 1966, with closer questioning, 21 patients out of 54 reported milder or stronger reac-

Table 4. *Lymphocyte transformation in patients with immediate and delayed allergy to insulin*

Pat.	Diagnosis	Duration of culture (days)	Transformed cells % bovine insulin				Reaction of intradermal skin test	
			without antigen	50 γ/ml	500 γ/ml	with PHA	immediate	delayed
1	Generalized urticaria	5	5.8	27.0	34.2	42.8	+	
2	after insulin injection	5	3.0	23.0	24.0	39.8	+	
3	Local delayed	5	3.0	13.0	14.3	49.0		+
4	allergic reaction	5	6.5	22.6	25.0	52.4		+
5	after insulin	5	2.0	27.0	29.1			+
6		5	2.5	14.0	14.9			(+)
7	Insulin-treated	5	4.0	3.0	4.0	58.6	∅	∅
8	diabetics	5	11.5	10.0	8.4	40.5	∅	∅
9	without allergy	5	4.6	7.0	7.6	50.2	∅	∅
10		5	18.0	13.5	14.8	39.6	∅	∅
11		5	6.7	6.2	9.3	∅	∅	∅
12	Non-diabetics	5	5.0	7.7	9.0	19.0	—	—
13		5	14.0	16.0	—	72.4	—	—
14		5	3.7	—	4.5	38.5	—	—
15		5	21.5	21.0	23.5	—	—	—
16		5	22.5	23.5	25.6	33.8	—	—

tions, either recently or earlier. In the literature the frequency of allergic reactions is said to be between 14% (ALLAN and SCHERER, 1932) and 55% (PALEY and TUNBRIDGE, 1952). If one applies particularly broad criteria, i.e. the slightest pain sensation even without cutaneous alterations, then one would expect a frequency approaching 55%. It is likely that the remainder of the patients undergo a subthreshold reaction of which they are unaware.

The question arises as to which critera permit the definition of a cutaneous reaction under observation as a true immune reaction of the delayed type (delayed hypersensitivity). The clinical picture corresponds to a delayed reaction in that pain and erythema develop in 8—10 or 12 hours, or even longer after the insulin injection. The true, delayed immune reaction is seen only after 24 to 36 hours. Thus the skin test provided a typical manifestation of delayed hypersensitivity in almost all patients: the observable maximum occurred after 24 hours. The histologic examination of the skin did not make a clearly positive contribution: 1. it could only be carried out on a few patients; 2. it yielded sometimes the typical picture of a delayed reaction and sometimes the picture of a granulomatous reaction in which the involvement of antibodies was not to be excluded. There remains the phenomenon of antibody formation by circulating blood cells. The direct antigen binding method is less well-known as a standard in-vitro technique to determine a delayed-type immune reaction, although it is frequently mentioned. Considering that the "Migration Inhibition Test" had at that time no application to patient testing, we have placed particular reliance upon direct antigen-binding. The subject has been studied recently by HEINEMANN and FEDERLIN (1969). TURK (1960) was able to observe direct antigen binding in the state of delayed allergy and used bovine serum albumin to sensitize lymphocytes; KAY and RIEKE (1963) employed fluorescein-labelled PPD. PELTIER and KOURILSKY (1966) demonstrated antigen fixation using human serum albumin and ov-albumin to sensitize cells, as already reported by STEFFEN and ROSACK in 1963. The cells used were always lymphocytes. The observations reported here: antigen binding to blood lymphocytes in patients at the onset of their delayed allergic reaction to insulin, have many parallels in experimental method. Much evidence suggests that this is a cellular immune reaction. The question remains as to why granulocyte-antigen binding is also demonstrated in several patients, especially in those with longer lasting allergic symptoms. Despite the negative outcome of investigations of the so-called cytophilic antibody, it may be that humoral antibodies are responsible, perhaps passively sensitizing the leukocytes, as observed by VAN ARSDEL and SELLS (1963) in allergic individuals (pollen-allergy). The observation that granulocytes may play a role in delayed hypersensitivity should not go unmentioned. Thus, WITTEN, WANG and KILLIAN (1963), studying the antigen binding of sensitized lymphocytes in humans with a positive PPD-skin reaction, expressed their opinion as follows: "We have the impression that neutrophils from positive skin reactors had a greater affinity for the antigen than the neutrophils from negative reactors." DE WECK and FREY (1966) observed the participation of various granulocyte forms in contact allergy. Furthermore, the work of STICKL and ENGELHARDT (1965) gives an impressive example of the existence of sensitized granulocytes, whereby leukocytolysis serves as an indication of specific reactivity to vaccinia virus after smallpox vaccination. Circulating leukocytes from vaccinated donors demonstrated the phenomenon of immunocytolysis after prolonged contact with the antigen, as shown by RICH and LEWIS (1928). Although the lymphocytes figured predominantly in this lysis phenomenon, granulocytes were unquestionably observed as well. MILLER and FAVOUR (1951) made the same observation in granulocytes of tuberculin-immunized mice. However, the participation of humoral antibodies paralleling the presentation of delayed hypersensitivity cannot be excluded, and must also be discussed in reference to the present investigations. Very recently ISHIZAKA, TOMIOKA and ISHIZAKA (1970) were able to demonstrate receptor sites for γG and γE in neutrophils and monocytes. While reaginic antibodies (γE) could not be demonstrated in the sera of our diabetics with delayed allergy to insulin, neutralizing antibodies (γG) were measurable in 8 out of 14 cases. The investigations on our own patients provided no clear answer to this question. In some, the determination of maximum insulin-binding capacity and demonstration of an insulin antibody coincided with the time of the delayed allergic reaction; in some it did not. These observations suggest a dissociation of the two immune reactions. Accordingly, it would be possible for the minute quantity of humoral antibody on the surface of cells to cause antigen binding, without being demonstrable with the techniques for serum antibodies. These questions, which remain open in respect to humans, should be satisfactorily answered in the subsequent investigations of guinea pigs.

The interpretation of delayed-onset allergic reaction to insulin in diabetic patients is essentially clarified by this observation from the realm of experimental immunology. DIENES and SCHÖNHEIT showed in 1929 that daily intracutaneous injections of small quantities of protein cause a mild delayed skin reaction in guinea pigs, occurring at the 3rd or 4th injection and changing on the 7th or 8th day into an Arthus phenomenon with the appearance of humoral antibodies. Similar observation were made by JONES and MOTE (1934) whose names have been appended to the delayed allergic phenomenon following small doses of protein. There exist certain distinctions in true delayed hypersensitivity, as propounded essentially by RAFFEL and NEWEL (1958). The Jones-Mote phenomenon occurs earlier than the true tuberculin reaction (after administration of the antigen) and it does not last as long as the latter. Thus there is little doubt this is a type of delayed hypersensitivity. It would exceed the scope of this paper to expound the details of this problem. The occurrence of delayed allergic reactions of the skin after minute quantities of protein — the Jones-Mote phenomenon — represents the best parallel to delayed allergy in diabetics.

8. Summary and Recommended Therapeutic Measures

Investigations of sensitized cells to insulin were successfully carried out utilizing immunofluorescence and immune adherence in 14 patients with a delayed local insulin-allergy. At the same time the serum of these patients was evaluated for humoral antibodies of the neutralizing and skin-sensitizing types. For 3 patients histopathologic preparations of the skin reactions were examined.

In every case the binding of insulin to circulating leukocytes was demonstrable by both techniques. Lymphocytes and granulocytes participated in the reaction. Initially in the delayed allergy to insulin the serum antibodies (via the passive hemagglutination method and the maximum insulin-binding capacity) could not be shown. The stage of delayed allergy preceded the demonstrability of humoral antibodies. In the later stages cellular and humoral antibodies of the neutralizing type coexisted. Skin-sensitizing antibodies (reagins) were found in only 2 patients with an immediate allergy to insulin. The allergic serum transfer test afforded proof of their presence.

The histologic examination of the skin biopsies yielded in part a clear delayed reaction and in part a hyperergic granulomatous reaction. Insulin binding to some of the cells of this inflammatory infiltrate was observed.

The results indicate that the delayed local allergic reaction after insulin injection is due to the sensitization to insulin and not to added substances. The reaction of immunologically competent cells with the antigen insulin is very probably effected by a cellular component of antibody nature — not, however, to be designated a cytophilic antibody. It seems to be produced by the sensitized cell itself. The delayed insulin allergy in humans resembles the Jones-Mote phenomenon occurring after repeated sensitization with small quantities of protein. This reaction belongs to the general category of specific cell-mediated hypersensitivity.

On the basis of these investigations in patients with a delayed localized insulin allergy, the following therapeutic measures can be recommended:

1. The occurrence of a mild local allergic reaction raises the question as to whether the insulin injection penetrates deeply enough into the subcutaneous tissue, since a superficial injection increases the tendency to allergy;

2. with correctly administered insulin injections, cutaneous reactions which do not exceed a moderate degree of intensity tend to regress spontaneously; thus, no change of insulin preparations is necessary;

3. where insulin allergy of greater intensity occurs, intracutaneous skin tests should be carried out with insulin of various species, and with the chemical substances with which the insulin is mixed (vehicles), to determine the true antigen. If such tests are not possible, the administration of insulin of another species should be tried (in general, this means a change from bovine to porcine insulin). If there is an allergic reaction to porcine insulin as well, the possibility that the skin reaction is induced by the acid pH of the insulin injection must be considered, and a rapid-acting neutral solution of pig insulin crystals may provide the solution as recommended by DECKERT and GRUNDAHL (Diabetologia 6, 15, 1970) to avoid antibody production.

4. Should an immediate localized reaction develop out of a delayed localized allergy, a generalized immediate reaction may be expected to follow. The insulin therapy should be discontinued, or continued under the strictest precautions with insulin of another species, since a cross-reaction to porcine insulin frequently develops in the immediate-type allergy to bovine insulin. The better course is to continue the treatment if possible, with sulfonylureas e. g. glibenclamid.

II. Investigations of Immediate Allergy to Insulin

Since the author's interest has largely been focused upon the pathogenic mechanisms underlying the delayed allergic reactions to insulin, only a few investigations have been done in patients with immediate allergic reactions. The main reason for this was to demonstrate reagin activity in the serum of those patients and thus to confirm the principal differences in pathogenesis between immediate forms of allergy insulin and delayed reactions.

One patient with immediate allergy to insulin (generalized urticaria) following a short period of delayed allergy to insulin has already been described (case history no. 8). Four other cases were observed.

Case History no. 15
W. V., 58-year-old male patient
Diabetes mellitus was diagnosed in 1940 and diet therapy was sufficient until 1950, but about 1950/51 insulin therapy was introduced. After the very first injection of insulin, generalized pruritus ensued. Therapy continued with 20 units depot insulin which led to minimal local skin reactions 1—2 hours after the injection, with occasional mild generalized pruritus. In subsequent weeks allergic manifestations increased: generalized urticaria, Quincke and glottal edema. Therefore insulin therapy was stopped and purely dietetic control continued until 1956, when an attempt at therapy with Invenol evoked severe colitis; again there was a return to dietetic control. In 1957 therapy was attempted with Long Insulin but discontinued after a few days because of severe generalized skin reaction. In the subsequent months administration of biguanides led to vomiting and bloody diarrhea, so was discontinued. In the following years attempts to treat the patient in different hospitals again involved insulin, sulfonylureas and biguanides, sometimes supported by antihistamines and cortisone preparations. In 1966 he was admitted to the Frankfurt clinic. The skin test showed severe immediate reaction to bovine and porcine insulin; no antigen-binding lymphocytes or granulocytes; serum reagins against both types of

insulin, as demonstrated by the AST test of LAYTON et al. (see Fig. 18). In the following weeks moderate therapeutic success was obtained with the administration of heated insulin according to DOLGER (1952) which apparently effected desensitization. Therapy was then continued with depot insulin 60 units (bovine) without appreciable allergic symptoms.

Summary. The patient showed immediate allergy to insulin, present since 1951, and based on the presence of reagins. No sensitized blood cells were demonstrable.

Subsequent History. After many months of insulin therapy without allergic manifestations, a most severe generalized allergy developed and the patient was admitted to an outlying hospital, where he died of lung embolism.

Case history no. 16

P. H., 32-year-old male patient

Diabetes mellitus was diagnosed in 1965 and treated with tolbutamide. In 1966 after a car accident he was admitted to an outlying hospital for surgical treatment. The change was made from tablets to insulin (32 U/day). After two days there were immediate local allergic reactions at the injection sites followed by generalized urticaria with anaphylactic shock on day 7. The hypersensitivity reaction was successfully treated with steroids and antihistaminics, insulin was withdrawn and therapy continued with sulfonylureas and phenformin. In autumn 1968 the glucose metabolism was found to be unbalanced, with increasing values of blood sugar. Therefore another attempt was made to employ insulin therapy which again was followed by a severe generalized urticaria. He was admitted to the university clinic of Ulm in December 1968. The skin test showed strong immediate reaction to all available insulins, no reactions to additives. Examination of peripheral white blood cells for binding of antigen with immunofluorescence and immune adherence showed 2% and 1% of reacting cells. Maximum insulin-binding capacity: 0.5 U/liter. Desensitization with small doses of insulin failed. Because of considerable overweight, he was treated with a low-calorie diet (600—800 Cal.) and glybenclamide and this led to a stabilized metabolism.

Case history no. 17

F. H., 43-year-old female patient

In 1964 diabetes mellitus was diagnosed and treated with carbutamide until 1967, then a change was made to Redul and biguanide. During March 1968 increased values were recorded for blood glucose and glucose excretion in the urine. Insulin therapy (bovine insulin) was started at 40 U/day. Nine days later, 1 hour after the injection of insulin, there was generalized urticaria and Quincke edema, treated with calcium, steroids and antihistaminics. The skin test showed strong immediate reaction (+ + +) against porcine insulin and similar (+ +) against bovine insulin, but no reaction to insulin additives. — Desensitization failed and the treatment was successfully continued with glybenclamide. An evaluation of peripheral white blood cells for antigen binding with immunofluorescence showed it to be less than 1%. (Immune adherence was not performed for technical reasons.)

Case history no. 18
M. B., 71-year-old female patient
In 1955 diabetes mellitus was diagnosed and therapy started with insulin (mixed: bovine-porcine), followed by local allergic reactions of the delayed type (onset 12—16 hours after the injection). Changing to other types of insulin was without effect on the dermal reactions, but balanced metabolism. Therapy continued with tolbutamide. Eleven years later the patient was admitted to an outlying hospital because of high blood glucose values. Beginning of insulin treatment was followed by local delayed allergic reactions during 4 days and by local immediate reactions for another 3 days. Then generalized urticaria and dyspnea led to withdrawal of insulin. Further trials with pure porcine or bovine insulin in frequent small doses had only transient success, so she entered the university clinic, Ulm. Blood sugar values were between 300 and 400 mg%, urine sugar 1.4%. The skin test showed severe reaction to all insulins (beef, pork, sheep) of the immediate type. No trial for desensitization was carried out because the metabolism was well balanced after treatment with glybenclamide. Immunocytology of peripheral white blood cells: Immunofluorescence 5%, immune adherence 3%.

Conclusion: Sera of two patients (cases 8 and 15) were examined for the presence of reagin activity with the allergic serum transfer test in monkeys according to LAYTON et al. (1965). Both showed strong positive reactions which could be abolished by heat inactivation. The sera of the other 3 patients in this group could not be tested because at that time no monkeys were available to the author and his coworkers.

In contrast to the positive results with sera of patients with immediate type allergy, the sera of all patients with delayed allergic reactions to insulin reacted negatively in the AST test. Obviously they contained no reagins, so that these cannot be responsible for the allergic reaction in these cases. — Lymphocytes of the peripheral blood did not bind antigen to a greater extent than cells of control persons. Thus, immediate type allergy and delayed type allergy to insulin can be distinguished sharply, not only by the clinical picture but also by the laboratory findings.

For recent findings in immediate type insulin allergy see: LIEBERMAN et al.: J. Amer. med. Ass. **215,** 1106 (1971).

III. Coexistence of Insulin Allergy and Insulin Resistance

Since the early days of insulin therapy, the synchronous appearance of insulin allergy and insulin resistance has been described many times (GLASSBERG, SOMOGYI and TAUSSIG, 1927; RUDY, 1931; GOLDNER and RICKETTS, 1942; SHERMAN, 1950; ENGBRING, ARKINS and LENNON, 1962). In these cases the diabetics suffer from localized or generalized allergy of the immediate type and, in addition, the insulin requirement necessary for stabilizing the glucose metabolism is much higher than normal. Skin-sensitizing antibodies and insulin-neutralizing antibodies are produced simultaneously. It is not known whether different antigenic determinants at the insulin molecule are responsible for both types of antibodies or whether the same chemical groups evoke antibody production in different clones of immunologically competent cells.

Another kind of connection may exist in patients in whom insulin allergy is followed by insulin resistance. SHIPP et al. (1965) found insulin allergy preceding insulin resistance in one-third of 34 cases. The allergy was of the immediate type, but some case histories gave no details about the allergy. The interval between insulin allergy and insulin resistance ranged from weeks to months and even years.

Very close relations existed between insulin allergy and insulin resistance in the cases described by KERP et al. (1965), FREI, CRUCHAUD and VANOTTI (1965) and FEDERLIN et al. (1966). In these patients a severe delayed allergic reaction to insulin developed during the first days of therapy. Positive delayed skin test, binding of antigen by sensitized blood lymphocytes and lack of serum antibodies to insulin were at that time regarded as the expression of delayed hypersensitivity to insulin. In the following course insulin-binding antibodies of the neutralizing type (in one case also of the skin-sensitizing type) developed more or less rapidly to very high levels leading to real insulin resistance. Both immune systems of the organism, i. e. immunologically competent lymphocytes and humoral antibodies, were stimulated simultaneously. One only can speculate whether these observations indicate an interdependence of the different immune systems, a hypothesis which in general has been abandoned by immunologists in favour of a theory postulating complete dissociation of delayed hypersensitivity and antibody production. Nevertheless, the observation mentioned above has been repeated in results with experimental animals. Insulin-sensitized guinea pigs with a clear-cut delayed hypersensitivity to insulin, if subsequently injected with the antigen (+CFA), later showed significantly higher titers of antibody than animals which developed only slight symptoms of delayed hypersensitivity to insulin. Thus, a marked phase of delayed allergic reactions to insulin at the beginning of therapy of diabetes mellitus should be taken as a warning to look out for insulin resistance.

D. Investigations of the Delayed Immune Reaction and Formation of Antibody to Insulin in Experimental Animals

The numerous difficulties encountered in evaluating the various immune reactions to insulin (insulin allergy, insulin resistance) under standardized conditions led us to carry out animal experiments. The intention was to produce a delayed immune reaction to insulin and then later to make a more exact study of the humoral antibodies in their varying stages. We hoped to be able to draw conclusions concerning insulin-treated diabetics from these results. The guinea pig was selected as the experimental animal, because this species, in contrast to numerous other kinds of animals, resembles man in its ability to reproduce a florid immune reaction of the delayed type as well as to produce humoral antibodies.

I. Investigations of the Delayed Immune Reaction to Insulin in Guinea Pigs

1. Material and Methods

a) Animals, Mode of Sensitization, Skin Test

400—500 g female albino guinea pigs (Pirbright-White breed) were employed. Fourteen days after subcutaneous sensitization with insulin in various concentrations (100—500 μg) together with complete Freund's adjuvant, an intracutaneous skin test was performed with 30 μg insulin. The outcome of the skin test was quantitatively measured by means of the Kröplin-Schnelltaster (see Fig. 25 a) for skin thickness. As a control, we measured the thickness of the skin on the contralateral side of the guinea pig's back after the injection of pure vehicle without insulin. The reading was made after 24 hours. An increase in skin thickness of more than 10 Kröplin units (1 Kröplin unit = 0.05 mm) was taken as positive, an increase of more than

20 Kröplin units as strongly positive. Animals with weaker skin reactions were excluded from further studies. In those fulfilling the criterion of a clearly positive delayed skin reaction, the following investigations were performed.

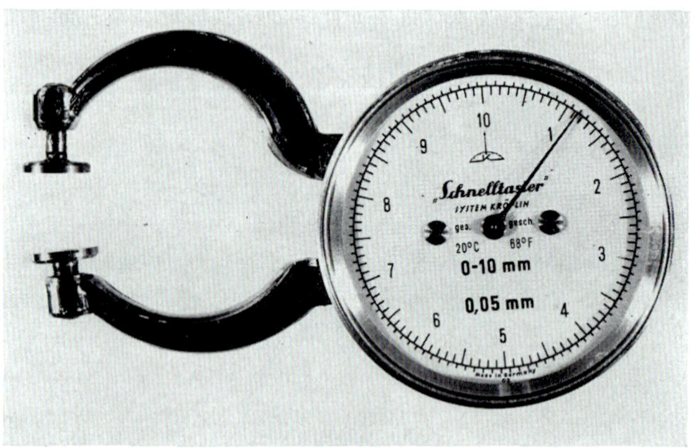

Fig. 25 a. Skinfold caliper (model Kröplin) for quantitative measurement of skin tests

b) Cytological Examination of Peripheral White Blood Cells

Antigen binding by lymphocytes was demonstrated by immunofluorescence (IF) and by immuno-cyto-adherence (ICA) according to Nota et al. (1964) as modified by Duffus and Allen (1969). The ICA was performed with insulin-coated sheep erythrocytes, bisdiazobenzidine being used as coupling agent.

The technique with white blood cells is essentially that already described in chapter C.I.2, where the separation of lymphocytes is obtained using glass wool. Since the lymphocytes of guinea pigs do not adhere well to glass surfaces, they were fixed onto slides by cell centrifugation according to Doré and Balfour (1965).

c) Transfer Test

Utilizing a cell filter, the lymph nodes from various regions of the body were fragmented and concentrated. The cells were concentrated in a quantity of 200×10^6 cells in Hank's solution to a total volume of 0.5 ml. This amount was injected intravenously into healthy guinea pigs of the same breed. In these recipients the same skin test as described above was carried out after 2 hours.

d) Migration Inhibition Test

Principle: Cells from the peritoneal exudate of sensitized animals were collected in glass capillary tubes, which were fixed to the bottom of small transparent chambers filled with culture medium. The antigen to be investigated is added to the medium in some of the chambers. While the exudative cells, consisting of approximately 80% macrophages and 20% lymphocytes, migrate in the form of a "cell tree" in the antigenfree chambers at 37° C, their proliferation is impaired by the presence of specific antigen. The extent of inhibition can be quantitatively determined by projection of the capillaries and by planimetric measurement of the surface formed by the migrating cells. The result is then compared with that for chamber preparations without antigen, giving the migration index:

$$\%\ \text{migration} = \frac{\text{planimetric value with antigen}}{\text{planimetric value without antigen}} \times 100.$$

The reaction between antigen and the sensitized lymphocytes in the exudate is responsible for the inhibition of migration. These cells release a soluble substance which impairs the mobility of the macrophages (BLOOM and BENNETT, 1968; DAVID, 1968). This "migration inhibition factor" in experiments performed with tuberculin is a protein with a molecular weight of approximately 68,000; it does not appear to be an antibody fragment.

The following substances were utilized as antigens: 1. the complete molecule of bovine insulin (i. e. the antigen employed for sensitization); 2. porcine insulin (to determine whether the sensitized cell is capable of cross-reacting); 3. isolated A and B chains of bovine insulin; 4. synthetic insulin fragments with amino acid sequences corresponding to portions of the B chain. We thank Dr. phil. nat. ROLF GEIGER of Farbwerke Hoechst AG for generously supplying these insulin fragments.

Technique:* 10 days after the injection of the antigen, 20 ml of sterile paraffin solution was given intraperitoneally to 20 experimen-

* The author thanks Dr. D. C. DUMONDE, Head of the Division of Immunology, Kennedy Institute of Rheumatology, London, for initiation into the technique and for helpful advice.

tal animals. Two days later the skin test (vide supra) was carried out and another 24 hours later the extent of cutaneous inflammation was quantitively measured from the skin thickness. After another 24 hours (i. e. on the 14th day after the injection of the antigen) the animals were placed in ether, bled via heart puncture and decapitated. The chambers were prepared according to the technique of DAVID et al. (1964): they were filled with an 85 : 15 mixture of guinea-pig serum and Eagle's medium, the latter including the antigen. The antigen concentration in the chambers varied from 30 μg/ml to 100, 300 and 900 μg/ml chamber medium. Then the laterally placed holes in the chamber were sealed with wax and the chambers placed in an incubator at 37° C. The first recording of macrophage proliferation was made at 5 hours, the last after 24 hours. This was effected by projecting onto a white surface the capillary tubes containing the washed-out cells (Zeiss projection microscope). The surface area was outlined and later evaluated quantitatively by means of a planimeter. The tests were carried out in three forms: sensitized cell with antigen in the medium; in control A the chambers contained sensitized cells but no antigen; in control B the chambers contained the exudative cells of unsensitized animals together with antigen in the medium. There should be no impairment of proliferation of the macrophages in either control.

e) Studies of Humoral Antibodies to Insulin

The serum of the sensitized guinea pigs was tested by the passive hemagglutination technique, and the binding capacity for ^{131}I-insulin was measured at intervals according to KERP et al. (1968) with the object of documenting the presence of insulin antibodies relative to the stage of the delayed immune reaction to insulin.

2. Results

An insulin dose of 400 μg injected into the foot pads with complete Freund's adjuvant proved to be the dose most effective in producing the state of delayed hypersensitivity to insulin. An intradermal skin test with 30 μg of antigen elicited a definite induration after 24 hrs (Fig. 25 b) and lasted until 48 hrs after the injection; this was not reproducible in the control animals. Only in those animals of the skin test groups with more than 10 Kröplin-units were further examinations undertaken.

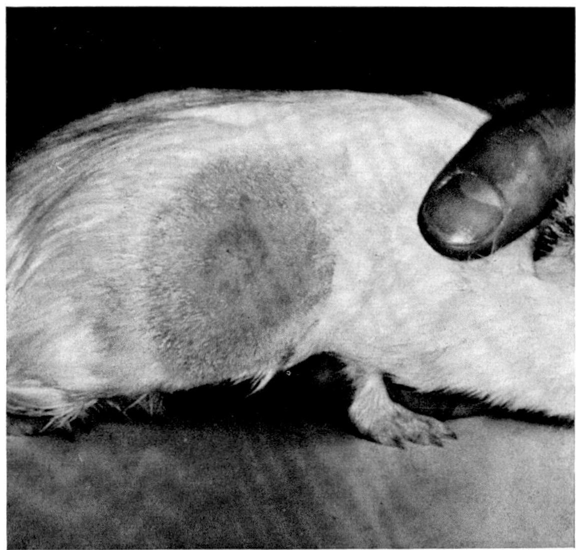

Fig. 25 b. Delayed skin reaction 24 hours after intradermal injection of 30 µg antigen in a guinea pig sensitized 14 days before with 400 µg crystallized bovine insulin

a) Cytological Investigations of the White Blood Cells

Antigen binding by sensitized white blood cells of the experimental animals was studied by immunofluorescence (FITC-insulin) and immunocytoadherence (ICA). The latter technique represents a modification to the immune adherence (IA) (according to Nelson, 1953) which was used in the study of insulin allergy in patients. While in IA the sensitized cells were incubated with complement, antigen and red cells, in ICA the red cells were already coated with insulin. In both instances adherence of the erythrocytes indicated antigen binding by the sensitized white blood cells. With immunofluorescence a distinct binding of the antigen by sensitized blood lymphocytes was observed in the guinea pig, similar to the state of delayed allergy to insulin in man. The microscopic picture was slightly different in that the fluorescence was less brilliant and there were fewer reacting cells (see Fig. 26). The percentage of specifically stained cells in the peripheral blood of 12 experimental animals reached a maximum of 5—6%, while less than 1% of the cells of 10 control animals showed binding of FITC-insulin. In another 7 experimental animals the percentage of antigen binding cells was not measurable for technical reasons (poor adherence of the cells to the

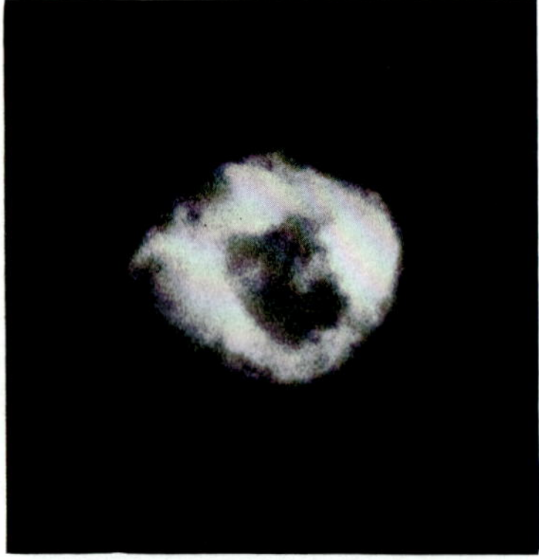

Fig. 26. Antigen binding (FITC-insulin) by a blood lymphocyte of a guinea pig with delayed allergic reaction to insulin. ×1400

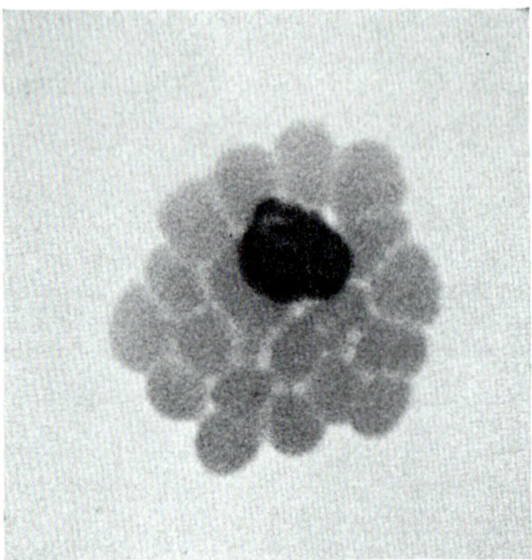

Fig. 27. Antigen binding by a lymphocyte of the same animal as in Fig. 26 with insulin-coated red cells of the same species (immuno-cyto-adherence). Triple-layer of red cells caused by the cytocentrifuge. ×1200

glass surface; weak and fuzzy staining of the sensitized cells). In contrast to this method, immuno-cyto-adherence, the second technique for demonstrating direct antigen binding onto the surface of sensitized cells, allowed much easier reading of the results, which were also clearly positive. An average of 8% of the white blood cells from 14 experimental animals showed adherent insulin-coated red cells, while this occurred only in 1% of cells of 10 control animals (Fig. 27). Further information and technical details are given in HEINEMANN, (1971).

b) Transfer Experiments

By injecting 200×10^6 lymph-node cells of sensitized animals, we were able to demonstrate the transfer of the delayed immune reaction in 9 guinea pigs. The skin test was carried out in the recipient

Table 5. *Transfer of delayed hypersensitivity to insulin in guinea pigs by means of lymph-node cells*

	Positive Transfer	Negative Transfer
A. experimental animals	9	6
B. control animals	0	9
type of transferred cells		
1. lymph-node cells	6	2
2. peritoneal exudate cells	1	5
3. spleen cells	1	4
4. lymph-node cells + peritone. exud. cells	3	1

animals 2 hours after the intravenous administration of these cells. In 6 animals the transfer did not succeed. Peritoneal exudate cells and spleen cells proved unsatisfactory for transfer. The results of the transfer experiments are in agreement with experience with other antigens in (non-inbred) experimental animals. The results are shown in Table 5 (from: FEDERLIN, KRIEGBAUM, and FLAD, 1968).

c) Migration Inhibition Test

The addition of 30, 100 and 300 µg insulin to the cellular preparation of peritoneal exudate from guinea pigs showed a statistically significant inhibition of migration on the basis of measured surface

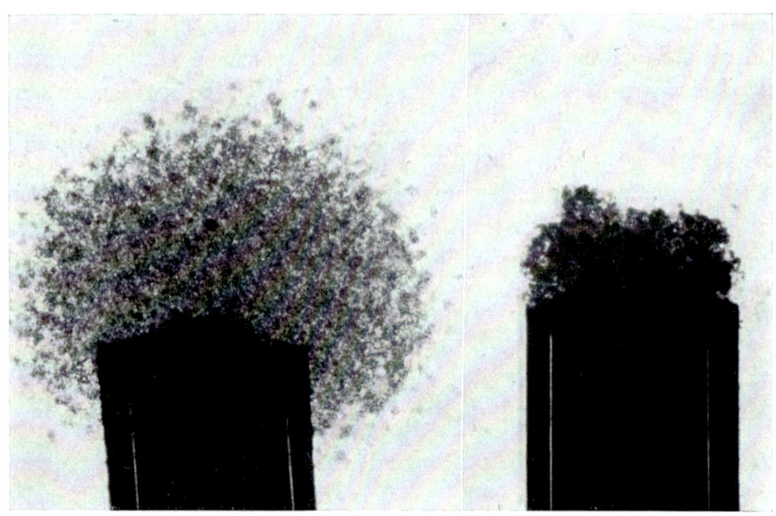

Fig. 28 a. Left: Normal migration of guinea pig peritoneal exudate cells in a chamber containing tissue culture medium alone. — Right: Migration inhibition of the cells of the same animal in presence of antigen

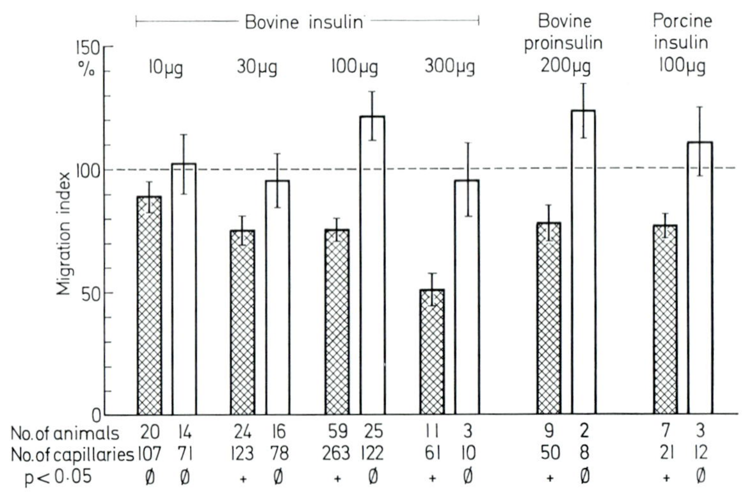

Fig. 28 b. Inhibition of macrophage migration (peritoneal exudate cells of insulin-sensitized guinea pigs) by the antigen in different concentrations (cross reaction with bovine insulin) and by proinsulin; hatched columns = cells of experimental animals; white columns = cells of control animals

area (preparations without antigen exhibit 100% migration). This is illustrated in Fig. 28 a and b. Thus these experimental animals had developed a delayed immune reaction whose intensity was proportional to the concentration of antigen in the chamber and was specific for the antigen involved. Migration was not inhibited when sensitized cells were incubated in the chamber medium without insulin nor when cells from unsensitized animals were incubated in the presence of insulin. In addition, the sensitized cells gave a cross reaction with the porcine insulin. An antigen dose of 10 μg in the chamber medium proved insufficient to evoke an inhibition of migration.

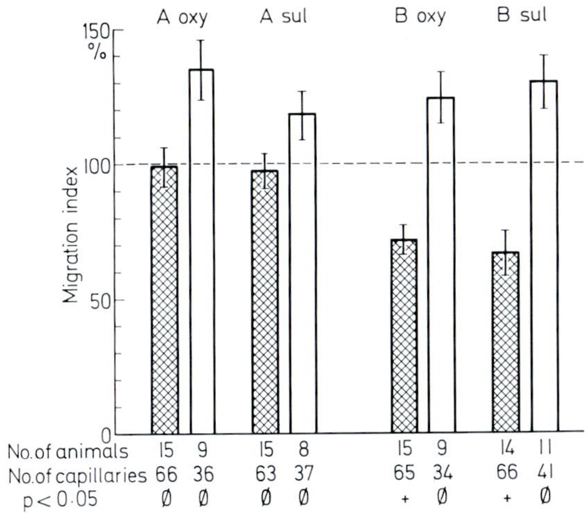

Fig. 29. Migration inhibition (cf. Fig. 28) by isolated A and B chains of insulin

Fig. 29 indicates the reactivity of lymphocytes which had been sensitized against the complete insulin molecule and were then incubated in vitro with isolated chains only. From these results it can be seen that the sensitized cells recognize only the antigenic configuration of the B chain. Incubation with the A chain evoked no statistically significant inhibition of migration.

In the experiments utilizing chain fragments (see Fig. 30) (synthetic fragments), only the fragment 03, corresponding to the amino acid sequence from no. 11 to no. 16 of the B chain, caused a statistically significant inhibition. With fragment 01, corresponding to the amino acid sequence 24 to 30 of the B chain, no inhibition was seen.

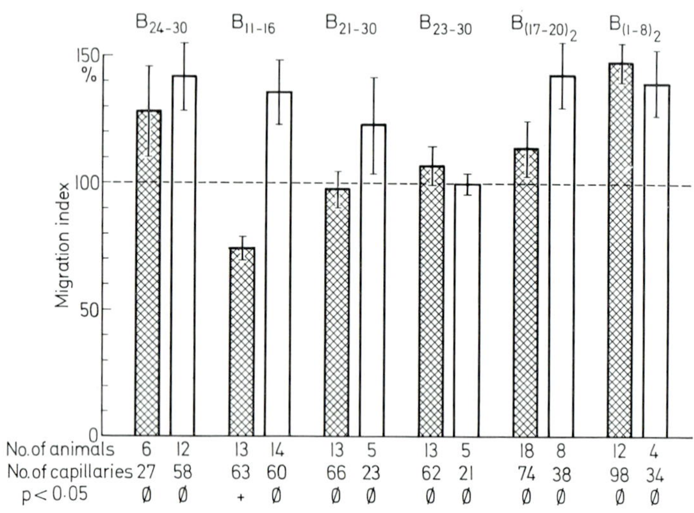

Fig. 30. Migration inhibition (cf. Figs. 28 and 29) by one synthetic insulin fragment of the B chain (B_{11-16}), no inhibition by other fragments

d) Humoral Antibodies

The investigations of the sera of sensitized guinea pigs by means of the passive hemagglutination technique indicated that the humoral antibodies were already present at the time when the animal had developed the definite capacity for delayed immune reactions. The results are summarized in Fig. 31 (HEINEMANN, KRIEGBAUM and FEDERLIN, 1969). Thus it is clearly shown that both types of immune reaction — delayed hypersensitivity and antibody formation — can appear apparently independently of each other. On the other hand, there appear to be interrelationships. For instance, there is a definite correlation between the intensity of the skin test and the formation of humoral antibodies. In extensive skin reactions the antibody titer was also quite high. Whether this might be the development of an

Arthus Phenomenon, which in actively immunized animals possibly is the result of a combined effect of sensitized cells and humoral antibodies at the site of injection of the antigen, must remain open to question.

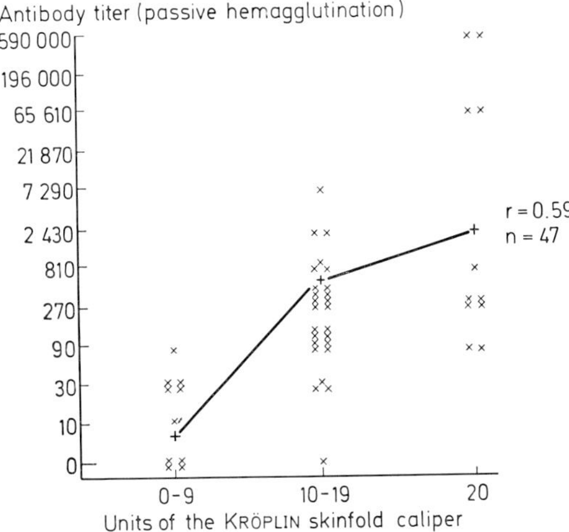

Fig. 31. Correlation between intensity of the skin reaction during the state of delayed hypersensitivity to insulin and antibody titer of the same animals after continued immunization. Animals with severe skin reaction produced the highest titers of antibodies

3. Discussion

The results have shown that a delayed immune reaction to insulin can be evoked in experimental animals (FEDERLIN et al., 1970; KRIEGBAUM and FEDERLIN, 1970). This reaction differs in the intensity of its course in individual animals but generally shows the criteria typical of this kind of immune reaction. The skin test produces a typical reaction after 24 hours which lasts for 48 or 72 hours. Also the positive outcome of the delayed immune reaction is confirmed. Further, the immune reaction was transferred to animals of the same species by means of lymphocytes. Finally, a direct binding of antigen onto the surface of sensitized cells was observed. The only other experiments of delayed hypersensitivity to insulin we found in the literature are those of Mc DEVITT (1963) and the recent publication of CLARK and MUNOZ (1970). These authors using the skin test as the tool for measuring delayed hypersensitivity observed similar results to our own. In desensitization experiments MUNOZ and CLARK found antigenic determinants on the isolated B chain but not on the A chain. Regarding their results obtained with humoral antibodies there is some disagreement. The authors did not observe reactivity between insulin antibodies and isolated chains and drew the conclusion that reactions between antibodies and the antigen insulin require conformational integrity of the molecule. This is in contrast to the findings of WILSON (1969) and to our own results (FEDERLIN and HEINEMANN, unpublished). By means of passive cutaneous anaphylaxis we were able to show that also isolated chains will react with antibodies which are directed against the complete molecule. Regarding delayed hypersensitivity reactions, our own observation of reactivity between a small fragment of the B chain corresponding to the amino acid sequence from no. 11 to no. 16 is of particular interest because according to the work of WILSON (1969) this specific area of the B chain is designated as immunologically insignificant. On the other hand with the fragment corresponding to the amino acid sequence 24—30 of the B chain no reactivity with sensitized cells was observed, although this region according to the experiments of WILSON contains an antigenic locus of the insulin molecule for humoral antibodies. While it seems to be clear that conformational integrity of the insulin molecule is necessary neither for interaction with circulating antibodies nor with sensitized cells, further research is needed to determine where the molecule contains antigenic loci accessible for only one or for both immune responses.

One must pose two questions: how far do these experimental models parallel the situation in insulin-utilizing diabetics who develop allergic manifestations? Is it possible to study this pathologic process by other means? Patients receive a daily subcutaneous injection of insulin, whereas in experimental animals the insulin is injected only once a week and then in combination with Freund's adjuvant. However, there is a certain parallel between the two kinds of sensitization in that the insulin is released only in small amounts from the emulsion with Freund's adjuvant. A possible parallel between animal and human conditions is that in both cases only certain individuals are subject to a particularly intense skin reaction. The same applies to antibody formation. As with diabetics, it was observed in individual guinea pigs that within a short space of time an increased production of insulin-neutralizing antibodies accompanied a strong reaction of the delayed type; this often led to insulin resistance. A fairly rapid sequence of intense delayed immune reaction and formation of humoral antibodies took place to the same extent in experimental animals as in diabetics. We thus held this to be the expression of an interrelationship between the two immune reactions, although on the other hand there is usually no temporal connection between them. Much argues for the concept that the first local, delayed onset skin reactions in insulin-treated diabetics be considered the expression of a transitional phase of a delayed allergy to insulin protein.

4. Summary

The sensitization of guinea pigs with 400 µg of bovine insulin together with complete Freund's adjuvant produced a local delayed skin reaction to insulin. The migration inhibition test performed on sensitized cells in in vitro conditions, as well as the positive transfer experiment and the direct binding of antigen onto the surface of sensitized cells, suggest the presence of a specific immune reaction of the delayed type against insulin. Coincident with the delayed immune reaction, the formation of insulin antibody could also be determined. High titers were achieved in some animals. In animals with an intense delayed skin reaction, it was observed that formation of humoral antibodies had already developed intensely. The statistical analysis yielded a clearly positive correlation.

II. Investigations of the Production of Humoral Antibodies

The first part of this paper has been concerned with immune cytology in the state of delayed allergy to insulin in man and in experimental animals; the second part will deal with the formation of anti-insulin antibodies in experimental animals. The species of choice was again the guinea pig, whose ability to produce antibodies to insulin is well known (literature in DECKERT, 1964).

These experiments were designed to determine 1. the fate of subcutaneously injected antigen and 2. the localization of humoral anti-insulin antibody formation. STEIGERWALD et al. (1960) had incidentally demonstrated the uptake of intravenously injected insulin by the liver. PARKER, ELEVITCH and GRODSKY (1963) had undertaken limited investigations of lymph nodes and spleen for anti-insulin antibody formation. More extensive studies of antigen and antibody production have not been done before. It was hoped that long-term antigen administration would supply the answers to two important questions:

1. Do glomerulosclerotic alterations of the Kimmelstiel-Wilson variety occur in experimental animals after prolonged administration of insulin?

2. Does insulitis occur in guinea pigs after injection of bovine insulin, as reported by RENOLD et al. (1964) for cattle and by the same group for sheep in 1969? GRODSKY et al. (1966) had been able to evoke experimental diabetes in rabbits by immunization with heterologous insulin.

It has been known for several years now that antibody production takes place not only in the stationary cells of the lymphatic system but in the circulating cells of the lymph and blood as well. Many and various observations have been made of the number of cells in the circulation having the ability to produce antibody; the variation depends greatly upon the choice of antigen for immunization and the choice of the method to provide evidence of antibody formation. Thus, for example, HULLIGER and SORKIN (1965) found evidence that up to 9% of all blood leukocytes in hyperimmunized rabbits were capable of antibody formation against human serum albumin. The technique employed was that of in vitro synthesis of antibody with radiochemical labelling. The use of the agar plaque technique according to JERNE and NORDIN (1963) or according to CUNNINGHAM (1965) yielded essentially lower values. We instituted studies of antibody formation by circulating blood cells after sensitization with insulin by means of plaque formation in agar by hemolytically active antibodies and insulin-carrying erythrocytes. The experiments were intended to indicate the presence of antibody-producing blood cells
1. before the appearance of humoral antibodies and
2. during hyperimmunization.

1. Material and Methods

a) Mode of Immunization

Guinea pigs weighing approximately 350—450 g were immunized with a mixture of crystallized bovine or porcine insulin (Hoechst AG) and complete Freund's adjuvant. For this, 15 mg insulin was dissolved in 10 ml distilled water and mixed in a homogenizer with complete Freund's adjuvant (Difco-LAB.) in a 1 : 1 proportion. This mixture was injected into the subcutaneous tissue between the scapulae of the guinea pigs. Each animal received 20 units of insulin. To prevent a hypoglycemic reaction, the animals were given sugared meal and sugared water. When signs of hypoglycemia developed, the animals received an additional subcutaneous injection of 10% glucose solution. The immunization was repeated at weekly intervals. After the 6th week the antigen alone, without Freund's adjuvant, was injected since in the interim sufficient granulation tissue had developed to permit a slower resorption of the insulin. Then after several weeks, or even months, Freund's adjuvant was again injected to stimulate antibody formation. Several animals were immunized for as long as 85 weeks. The long-term immunization was done with porcine insulin.

b) Detection of Antibody-forming Cells in the Peripheral Blood

α) Isolation of Blood Cells

A heart puncture was performed daily up to the third week in two guinea pigs; the 4 ml of blood obtained were then mixed with heparin at 50 units/ml. The blood was drawn up in a hematocrit tube and centrifuged in the cold at 2000 rpm for 8 minutes. The erythrocytes sedimented out initially and the leukocytes formed a small overlying white stratum (the Buffy coat). These were pipetted out and suspended in a citrate-saline solution (100 ml 3.8% Na citrate/ 1000 ml physiological saline). The centrifuged cells were later adjusted to a concentration of 10^6 cells/ml in normal Eagle medium. The leukocyte spreading could be enhanced by the addition of Dextran 250 to heparinized blood according to the method of SKOOG and BECK (1956). In the hyperimmunized animals two such tests were performed between the 40th and the 60th injection of antigen.

β) Plaque Technique (According to CUNNINGHAM*)*

In the technique according to CUNNINGHAM (1965) normal 2 × 2 cm glass slides are twice layered with a 7 μ thickness of paraffin. From the center a circle 1 cm in diameter is cored. 0.05 ml of the leukocyte suspension is added to the cored-out chamber in the paraffin layer together with 0.05 ml of a suspension of sheep erythrocytes in Eagle medium (concentration 10^9/ml) and with 0.05 ml of guinea-pig serum diluted 1 : 5 with Eagle medium; this is done at 0° C. The cell mixture is closed over by a coverslip so that excessive cells and fluid can be drawn outward with filter paper. The rim of the coverslip is then sealed with beeswax. The slide is then incubated at 37° C. The first plaques can be seen after 1 to 2 minutes; the maximum formation occurs after 20 minutes and further incubation does not increase it. The plaques are counted using a phase-contrast microscope (Zeiss). The results are given as plaques/100,000 white cells. At higher magnification the lysed erythrocytes are recognizable as ghost cells within the plaques; the center of such a plaque contains a white blood cell. The sheep erythrocytes are there to serve as indicators for the presence of antibody in the white blood cells and are therefore previously treated with insulin as follows: the red cells are obtained by venopuncture (vena jugularis); 100 units heparin/10 ml whole blood are added to prevent coagulation. After sedimentation the erythrocytes are twice washed with phosphate-buffered saline. Then 1 ml of the erythrocyte sediment is suspended in the following solution: 5 ml physiological saline, 5 ml double isotonic phosphate buffer (pH 7.4), 10 ml tannic acid solution (5 ml tannic acid/40 ml physiologic saline). This suspension is kept for 10 minutes in a water bath at 37° C and then centrifuged at 2000 rpm for 2—3 minutes. The erythrocyte sediment is again washed with 10 ml phosphate-buffered saline. 15 mg bovine insulin (Hoechst AG) is dissolved in 5 ml distilled water with the addition of a small portion of 1 N HCl (wetted glass stirring rod). Then 10 ml of doubly isotonic phosphate buffer (pH 7.2) is added. A suspension of 6 ml physiological saline, 12 ml insulin solution and 0.25 ml of the tanned erythrocyte sediment is used to coat the erythrocytes. This mixture is well shaken and then kept at room temperature for 20 minutes. Afterwards the suspension is centrifuged at 2000 rpm for 4 minutes and the sediment is washed according to the method of ARQUILLA and STAVITSKY (1956) with 3.5 ml of 1% (inactivated) sheep serum.

Complement preparation and complement absorption: a heart puncture is performed on normal guinea pigs. The fresh blood is kept at 4° C until the clot has separated from the serum. The clotted blood is centrifuged in the cold and the fresh serum is frozen at – 30° C in 0.5 ml portions. Since guinea-pig serum contains naturally-occurring antibodies to erythrocytes of various species (rabbits, sheep, man), these are absorbed onto sheep erythrocytes according to the technique of CUNNINGHAM to prevent an unspecific reaction. Thus sheep erythrocytes are thrice washed with physiological saline and centrifuged at 3000 rpm for 5 minutes. 1 ml of packed erythrocytes is incubated with 20 ml normal guinea-pig serum in an ice bath for 5 minutes; then the mixture is centrifuged in the cold centrifuge at -2° C at 3000 rpm for 10 minutes. The supernatant is pipetted off and the erythrocytes are removed. The serum is then resuspended in the same manner with fresh erythrocytes and the absorption is repeated 5 times in this fashion. After the third absorption a test is made to evidence the presence of natural antibodies. Thus a 2.5% erythrocyte suspension in Wallace-Mayer buffer is prepared. 0.5 ml of this suspension is incubated with 0.1 ml normal guinea-pig serum for 60 minutes at 37° C. The suspension is then abruptly centrifuged. A clear supernatant confirms that the natural antibodies to erythrocytes have been eliminated. If hemolysis is present, then the absorption must be continued.

To be certain that complement with adequate hemolysing qualities was present for these investigations, the serum of 15 guinea pigs was mixed and complement activity was titrated according to the method of GIGLI (1966). (For details see FEDERLIN, BIEDERMANN and PFEIFFER, 1969.)

For control purposes, the chamber was filled with the following variations: without complement; red cells without insulin coating, without leukocytes, without leukocytes but with additional active guinea-pig anti-insulin serum, in order to determine whether the erythrocytes contained adequate insulin.

c) Binding of ^{131}Iodine-labelled Insulin

While in patients with insulin antibodies the maximum insulin-binding capacity of the serum was measured, anti-insulin sera of immunized guinea pigs were examined by definition of the titer (dilution of serum) which binds a definite amount of ^{131}iodine-labelled insulin.

Principle: Different dilutions of antiserum were added to 1 mU ^{131}I insulin and the amount of antiserum capable of binding 50% of the antigen was measured, i. e. 500 μU ^{131}I insulin. The result is known as the titer of the antibody.

Technique: The technique was performed, with slight differences, according to KERP, STEINHILBER and KASEMIR (1966).

d) Passive Hemagglutination (for Technique see Paragraph C.I.5.a.β)

e) Immunohistological Techniques

4 days after the last insulin injection the animals were given an ether narcosis and bled by heart puncture. Directly afterwards the following tissues were removed: 1. granulation tissue from the area of the insulin injection, 2. locally draining lymph nodes, 3. spleen, 4. bone marrow, 5. liver, 6. kidney, 7. pancreas. The tissue portions obtained were immediately frozen in a 10 ml glass tube to $-90°$ using CO_2-acetone mixture and subsequently kept deep frozen at $-30°$. One half of the pancreas was fixed for 12 hrs in formalin and embedded in paraffin.

In further processing, the frozen tissue was thawed and then immediately sectioned with the cryostat. From the lymphatic organs touch-preparations were also made. Section and touch-specimens were fixed for 30 minutes in 95% alcohol and then dried, according to the method of PARKER, ELEVITCH and GRODSKY (1963).

To localize the antigen in the tissue, we employed FITC-labelled anti-bovine and anti-bovine insulin antibodies (the globulin fraction) of guinea pigs. For control purposes, we covered the tissue with a dye-containing normal guinea pig serum and with a labelled anti-guinea-pig serum from sheep. Also the inhibition technique was used whereby the binding of the labelled antibody is blocked after pre-incubation of the tissue with an unlabelled antibody. Labelled antigen (FITC-insulin) was used to localize the insulin antibodies. The controls consisted of layering of the preparations with FITC-labelled bovine serum albumin, with free dye as well as the use of the inhibition technique (preincubation of the specimen with unlabelled insulin which then later blocks the binding of the labelled hormone).

f) Histological Techniques

The remaining portion of the kidney obtained was fixed in 4% Formalin while for the pancreatic tissue a medium according to SUSA for 4—6 hours (70 cc Susa solution + 30 cc 30% formalin) was used. Usually the formalin-fixed tissue was embedded in paraffin after methyl benzoate treatment, but the pancreas was embedded in Cremolan (polyethyleneglycol 1.500).

The tissues embedded in paraffin were stained with hematotoxylin — eosin, and the renal tissue with elastica — VON GIESON (ROMEIS, 1948) as well as with Congo red (ROMEIS, 1948).

For selective staining of α and β cells of the islets of Langerhans in the Cremolan-embedded pancreas tissue, we employed the following method for which we are indebted to Dr. BÄNDER (Hoechst):

Imbedding

1. Fixation of the pancreas in Susa mixture 8—15 hours
2. alcohol 70% bath (2—3 times each 4—5 hours)
3. absolute alcohol: 1 hour
4. benzol: 30 minutes
5. absolute alcohol: 1 hour
6. Cremolan I: 8—12 hours
7. Cremolan II: 2—3 hours
8. Cremolan III: 2—3 hours
9. rinse with fresh Cremolan
10. embedding

Preparation of the Cremolan sections: the glass slides are finely layered with a mixture of:

1 part serum albumin 10%
1 part glycerin
a few grains of camphor

and allowed to dry for a few days. The sectioned tissue is dropped on to the moist slides, then allowed to dry for several hours.

Staining

1. Absolute alcohol 10 minutes
2. Lugol's mixture 10 minutes
   (1 part Lugol's solution, 1 part 70% alcohol until the formation of a red-brown cognac-colored-solution).
3. Sodium thiosulfate 0.5% 10 minutes
4. Brief washing in water 2—3 times
5. oxidation approximately 2 minutes
   in a mixture of
   distilled water 70 cc
   H_2SO_4 5% 20 cc
   $KMnO_4$ 2.5% 20 cc
6. bleach in sodium bisulfate 5% very briefly until the section is decolorized. This solution must be always freshly prepared.
7. Brief washing in water 3—4 times
8. alcohol 70%: 1 minute

9. aldehyde fuchsin: 2 hours
10. absolute alcohol: briefly
11. tap water: briefly
12. nuclear staining with
    iron trioxyhematein (Hansen): 5 minutes
13. Rinse with water: 20 minutes
14. distilled water: 1—2 minutes
15. counterstain with
    Patent blue-orange G: 20 minutes
    (preparation of stain vide infra)
    Lay the slides on a level surface and cover with the stain.
16. Alcohol 70%: briefly submerge 5 sec.
17. absolute alcohol: briefly submerge 5 sec.
18. solution I Acetone 70 cc, Benzol 30 cc } briefly submerge 5 sec.
19. solution II Acetone 30 cc, Benzol 70 cc } briefly submerge 5 sec.
20. solution III Acetone 5 cc, Benzol 95 cc } briefly submerge 5 sec.
21. benzol: briefly submerge 5 sec.
22. Xylol
23. Cover with Eukitt

Preparation of the Patent blue-orange G Solution
Solution I: 800 mg Patent blue VF in 100 ml water
Solution II: 800 mg Patent blue AE
1 g phosphotungstic acid in 100 ml water
Solution III: 600 mg Orange G
1 g phosphotungstic acid in 100 ml water

Solution I 1 part: Solution II 1 part: Solution III 2 parts:	This mixture must always be freshly prepared before use as separately each substance remains stable longer.

The imprint preparations obtained from lymphatic tissue (lymph nodes and spleen) by extirpation or even from frozen tissue are stained with Giemsa solution as described by Romeis (1948):

1. Place the sections in distilled water; change once
2. thinned Giemsa solution (1 : 100 with distilled water): 2 hours

3. wash in distilled water
4. differentiate and dehydrate in
   a) acetone 95 cc
      xylol 5 cc
   b) acetone 70 cc
      xylol 30 cc
   c) acetone 30 cc
      xylol 70 cc
   d) xylol
5. cover with Eukitt

2. Results

a) Antibody-forming Cells in Blood

The attempt to investigate blood cells by taking samples from the same animal daily after the administration of antigen failed. Since enough blood could be obtained only by heart puncture, the animals died after the 4th, 5th, 6th or 7th puncture. Daily blood withdrawal was successful in two new animals (a total of 90 for this experiment) which had been immunized at the same time. A portion of the blood was mixed with heparin to obtain cells for the cytological investigations; the remainder was kept for the serum to be used for the passive hemagglutination test.

The existence of antibody-producing and antibody-secreting cells in blood after insulin sensitization is demonstrated by the following findings. In the small chambers prepared according to the instructions of Cunningham (1965) there appeared certain white blood cells in the proximity of which erythrocytes labelled with insulin could be lysed. Observation with the phase contrast microscope at low magnification revealed dark plaques within the field of cells. At high magnification it could be seen that in the center of such a plaque a mononuclear leukocyte lay surrounded by so-called "ghost" erythrocytes (Fig. 32). The forms of the lysed cells, i. e. the stroma of the erythrocytes, impaired the local movement of the adjacent intact erythrocytes and therefore permitted the plaques to remain in the chamber after 48 hours. The size of these areas remained the same within narrow limits.

For the most part only the first and second row of adjacent erythrocytes were lysed, rarely the third or fourth. The diameter at the middle of a plaque was 30—40 μ. The external appearance (mononuclear) and the cell diameter (6—8 μ) indicated that the central cell was a lymphocyte or at least a lymphoid cell, not, however, a monocyte. In the vicinity of segmented granulocytes no plaques were seen. The result of the calculations of the 10 chambers per blood test

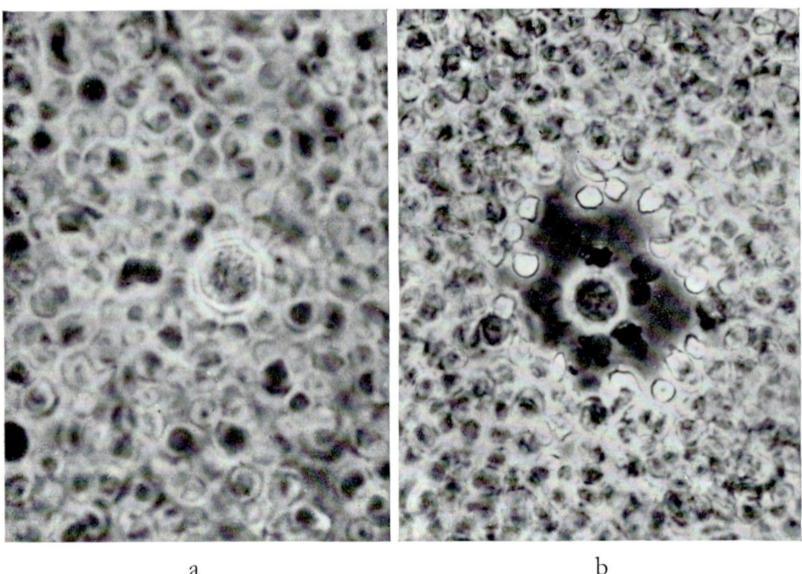

Fig. 32. Right: Demonstration of release of insulin antibodies by a mononuclear blood cell with the plaque technique according to CUNNINGHAM (1965). a Control with uncoated red cells; b Lysis of insulin-coated red cells in presence of complement. ×500

is shown in Table 6. This represents the number of plaque-forming cells/100,000 blood leukocytes in each of the two animals injected once weekly with antigen over 6 weeks. These results indicate that two days after the first administration of antigen a few antibody-producing cells appeared in the peripheral blood, this number being further increased on the 3rd day, reaching its maximum on the 4th day. On the 5th and 6th days the number declined. On the 7th day no plaque-forming cells were to be found in the blood. In contrast, after the second immunization the plaque-forming cells were already found on the first day; the number increases on the second day after the injection, reaching its maximum on the 3rd day. Despite minor differences, both animals evidenced the same phenomenon. After the 4th day the number of cells decreased and on the 6th or 7th day after the second immunization practically no plaques could be found. After the third immunization plaque formation again occurred on

Table 6. *Number of plaque-forming cells per 100 000 blood leucocytes in pairs of animals after weekly immunization with insulin*

Days after immunization	1st week		2nd week		3rd week		4th week		5th week		6th week	
1	0	0	5	1	3	4	2	3				
2	1	1	11	7	9	12	3	3				
3	5	11	21	19	5	7	5	5	1	3	0	2
4	23	27	7	7	3	5	2	3	0	0	0	0
5	5	7	4	4	1	1	1	2				
6	2	2	0	1	0	1	1	0				
7	0	0	0	0	0	0	0	0				

Table 7. *Appearance of humoral antibodies to bovine insulin in guinea pigs after weekly injection of insulin, detectable with passive hemagglutination*

Days after immuni-zation	1st week		2nd week		3rd week		4th week		5th week		6th week	
1	—	—	—	—	—	—	90	270	270	810	270	90
2	—	—	ϕ	ϕ	30	30	810	810	810	810	810	810
3	—	—	—	—	—	—	810	810	2430	810	810	2430
4	ϕ	ϕ	ϕ	ϕ	810	810	7290	7290	7290	2430	2430	21870
5	—	—	—	—	—	—	7290	7290	196830	21870	2430	21870
6	ϕ	ϕ	30	30	—	—	—	—	65310	21870	2430	7290
7	—	—	—	—	—	—	—	—	—	—	—	—

the 1st day, becoming more obvious on the 2nd day. These values however were never as pronounced as the maximum values achieved during the first two weeks. On the 3rd day the plaque-forming cells decreased in number and by the end of the 3rd week only a few remained. A similar pattern was seen after the fourth administration of antigen. In the 5th and 6th weeks afterwards the antibody-producing cells were very infrequently found. After the fourth administration values reached only the maximum seen in the control animals (2—3 plaques/100,000 leukocytes). The results of the serum antibody measurements of the same animals are shown in Table 7. The temporal relationship between the appearance of antibody-producing cells and the titer of humoral antibodies to insulin indicates clearly that the decrease in the number of these antibody-producing cells in the blood is associated with the increase in serum humoral antibodies (Fig. 33). Further measurements of insulin antibodies in guinea pigs will be discussed in the following chapter.

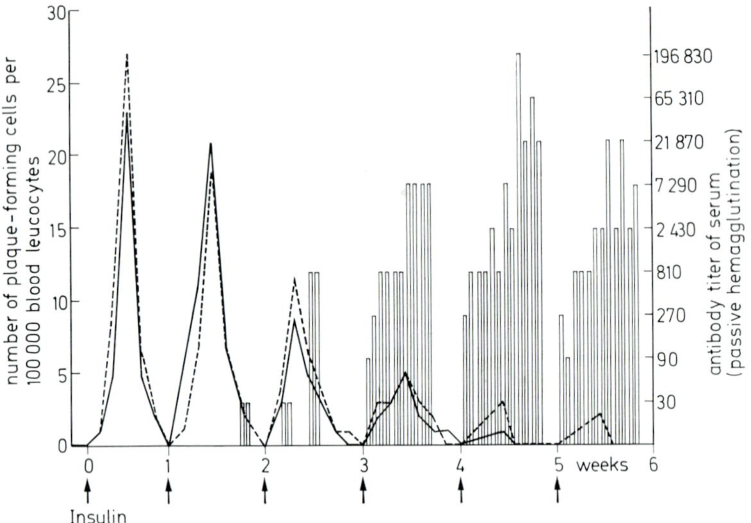

Fig. 33. Appearance of antibody-forming cells and of humoral antibodies in the peripheral blood after several injections of insulin + CFA

b) Humoral Antibodies

α) Binding of ^{131}Iodine-labelled Insulin

The binding of ^{131}I insulin by guinea-pig anti-insulin serum was measured mainly in order to see whether passive hemagglutination can detect small amounts of antibody, especially during the first period of antibody formation. Furthermore the two methods should be compared in high dilutions of antisera.

As can be seen in Fig. 34, passive hemagglutination is less sensitive in detecting small amounts of antibodies than the method with radioactive insulin. Sera with HAG-titers ranging from 1 : 10 to 1 : 270 exhibited similar binding of ^{131}I insulin as sera with a titer of 1 : 810. On the other hand sera with positive hemagglutination in very high

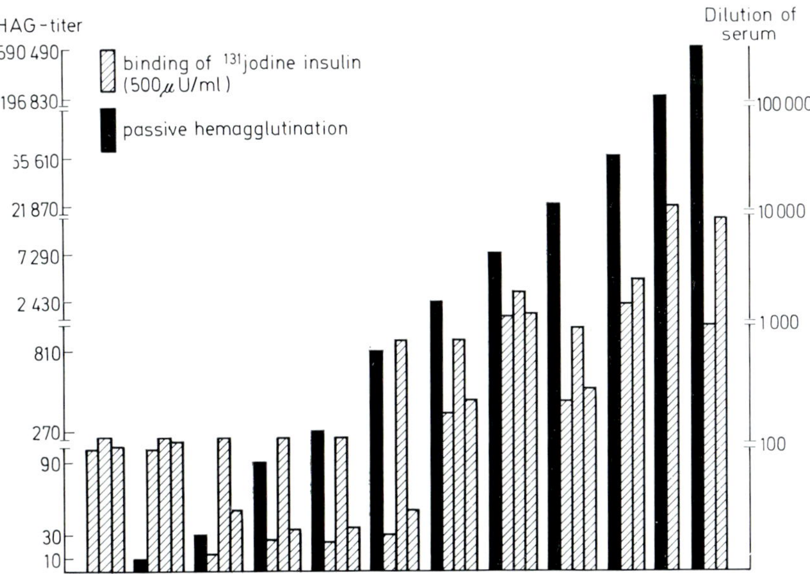

Fig. 34. Comparison of the insulin antibody titer obtained with passive hemagglutination and with binding of ^{131}I insulin

dilution (1 : 490,000) showed "relatively" low binding of the radioactive insulin. It remains an open question whether this expresses different types of antibodies. Furthermore, the amount of insulin on the surface of red cells is less exactly defined than the dose of ^{131}I insulin added to the reaction mixture. In general, with the exception of low titers, there is a rough parallel between the results obtained with both techniques. The binding of 500 μU ^{131}I insulin of a 1 : 10,000 diluted serum, i. e. binding of 5 U/ml, demonstrates the high concentration of antibodies in a serum with an HAG titer of 1 : 590,490.

β) Passive Hemagglutination

By means of the passive hemagglutination test, antibodies were detectable in small quantities after the second immunization and even at the end of the second week. The titer increased further in the 3rd and 4th weeks and attained its maximum after the fifth immunization. The results are given in Fig. 35. In the majority of animals

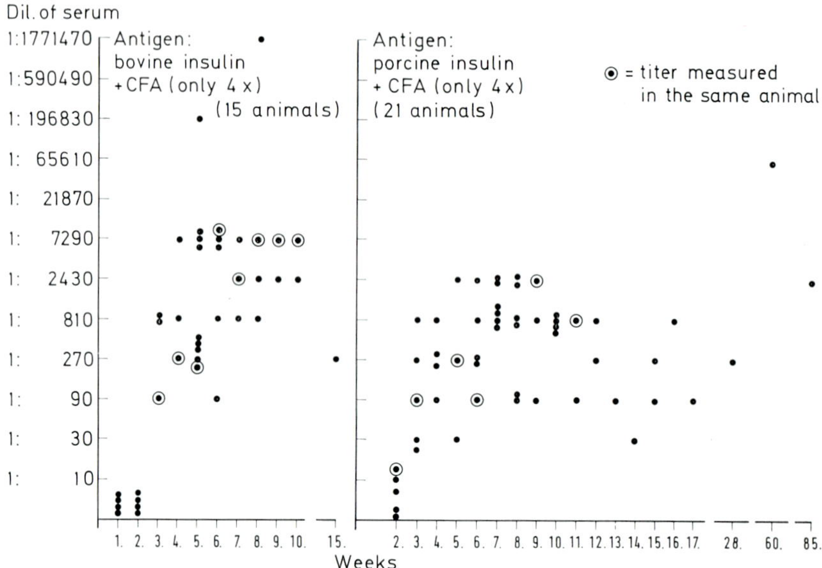

Fig. 35. Antibody titer of guinea pigs after weekly immunization with bovine and with porcine insulin (+CFA). Passive hemagglutination

the titer did not increase after the 6th week although the antigen administration was continued in weekly intervals. Only in a few animals were higher titers reached, implying particularly active antibody formation.

To study the effect on the formation of antibody of antigen injections at longer intervals, in some animals the second insulin injection was given after 4 weeks and the animals were bled 14 days later. As shown in Fig. 36, this type of immunization markedly enhances antibody production. Therefore this schedule of immunization is much more suitable for inducing active antibody formation;

however, this was not the objective of the present study. On the contrary, guinea pigs should be immunized regularly, and without breaks, as in human diabetics.

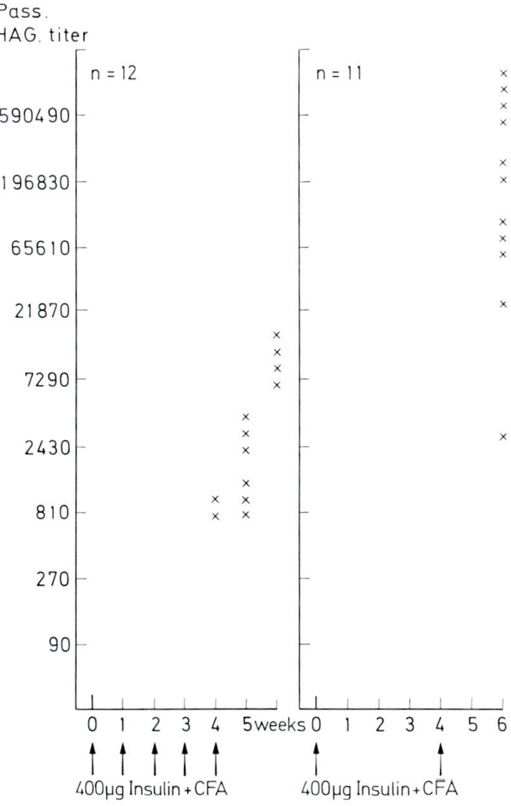

Fig. 36. Titer of insulin antibodies in guinea pigs produced by different immunization procedures (passive hemagglutination)

A sample of guinea pigs immunized against porcine insulin had on the average one titer less activity compared with animals injected with bovine insulin. It seems reasonable to conclude that in guinea pig bovine insulin is more immunogenic than porcine insulin. But the lower titer could also be the result of the variable concentration of antigen in the reaction medium, because it is not possible to label the erythrocytes with antigen for more than a few days (FRASER and

HARTOG, 1962). Nevertheless, differences in antigen loading of the erythrocytes are compensated for by the frequent performance of the technique.

γ) Binding of Insulin in Pancreatic Tissue

The ability of an antibody to react with insulin can be assessed by means of the immune histology of the pancreas. Here the insulin antigen is found in situ, and what has to be determined is not the binding of antibody to extracted insulin but to insulin at its site of formation. In these investigations good agreement was found between the level of antibody titer as measured by the passive hemagglutination technique and the demonstrability of insulin in the beta cells of the islets of Langerhans. Labelling with fluorescein isothiocyanate (FITC) permitted excellent demonstration of insulin in beta cells with high-titer serum in cryostat sections as well as in formalin-fixed pancreas while low-titer serum showed no specific staining (Fig. 37 and 38). The labelling of these sera could be held approximately the same intensity, the F/P ratio ranging between 1.0 and 1.5.

With a high-titer serum against bovine insulin, the pancreas of different animal species were investigated to compare the demonstrability of the beta cells. The results were as follows:

man	rat	mouse	guinea pig	rabbit	calf	beef	pig	sheep
+	++	++	+	++	+++	+++	+	++

+ weak,
++ medium,
+++ brilliant immunofluorescence of beta cells

The weak fluorescence of the beta cells in man is most probably caused by the fact that only autopsy specimens could be examined, and autolytic processes may have altered the insulin or influenced the immunohistological reactions for other reasons. The distinct but weak reaction with insulin of the beta cells of guinea pigs may be due to the large difference in the composition of amino acids in insulin as between the bovine and guinea pig species which affects 18 positions. The primary structure of insulin of the other species is much more closely related to beef insulin which was used as antigen.

Nevertheless, the phenomenon of the binding of guinea pig antibodies against heterologous insulin to the insulin in the pancreas of the same species (Fig. 39) is an interesting observation because blood

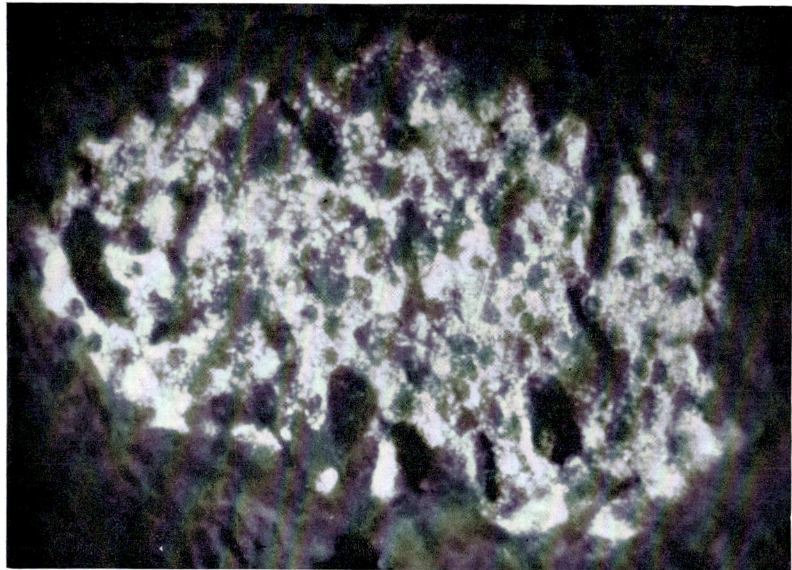

Fig. 37. Immunohistological demonstration of insulin in β-cells of an islet of Langerhans of the rat. Cryostat section. Direct immunofluorescence: FITC-labelled antibody (globulin fraction) of the guinea pig against bovine insulin. ×480

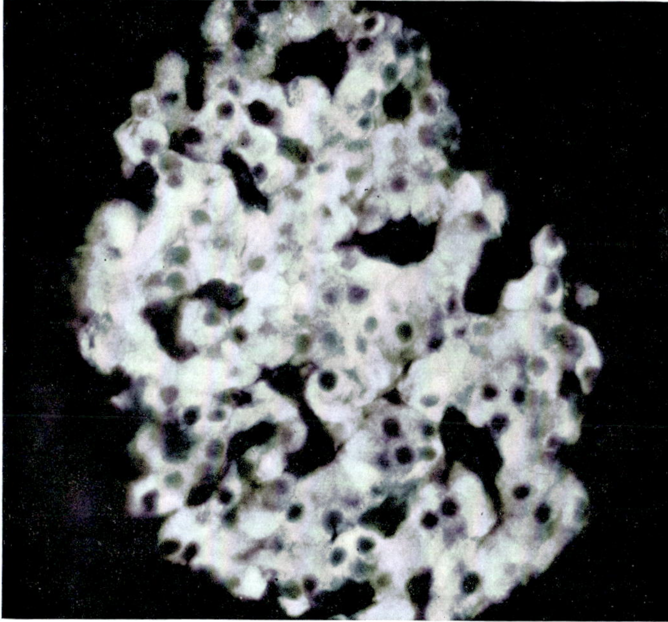

Fig. 38. Same conditions as in Fig. 37, but pancreas fixed in formalin and embedded in paraffin. ×480

sugar and urine sugar controls in the experimental animals at different times during the immunization gave no indication that endogenous insulin was neutralized by these antibodies with the consequent induction of a diabetic syndrome.

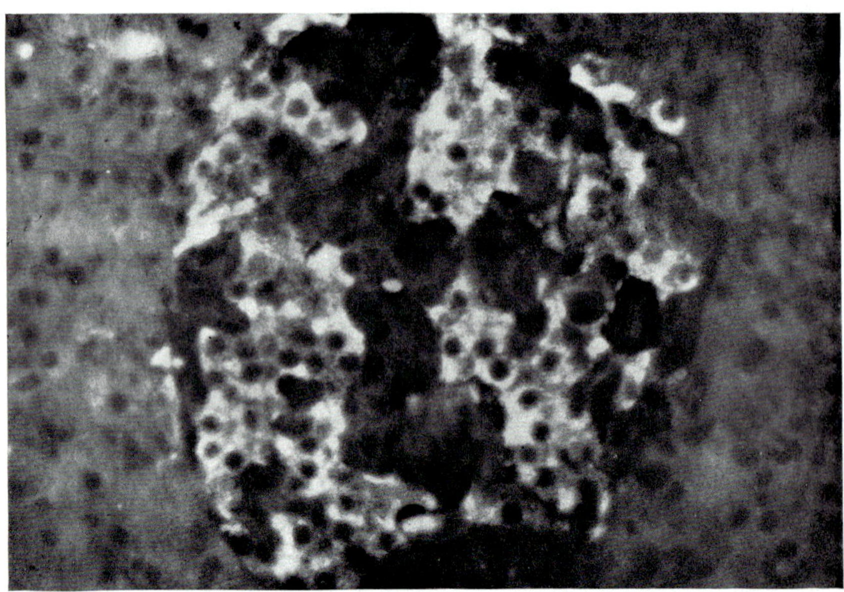

Fig. 39. Immunofluorescent staining of an islet of Langerhans in the guinea pig with an FITC-labelled guinea pig antibody against bovine insulin. Formalin fixation, paraffin embedding. ×480

δ) The Effect of Labelling with FITC on the Immunological Properties of Insulin and Insulin Antibodies

Regarding insulin, ARQUILLA, OOMS and FINN (1966) showed that careful labelling with FITC — in contrast to labelling with radioactive iodine — produced essentially no alteration of the immunological properties. To our knowledge, there have been no reports on whether the activity of insulin antibodies is reduced after labelling with FITC. In these investigations the influence of the dye was tested with the passive hemagglutination. The labelled insulin had an F/P ratio of 0.1—0.5 (as maximum) i. e. was weakly labelled; the F/P ratio of the insulin antibodies ranged between 1.0 and 1.5. Insulin and insulin antibodies were tested in either the unlabelled or labelled state.

FITC-labelled bovine and porcine insulin showed no reduction in their immunological properties as compared with the unlabelled antigen, i.e. the titer remained unchanged. In contrast, when labelled antibody was tested with unlabelled antigen, a decline in titer was observed. The loss of antibody activity ranged between one and two dilution steps (titers of hemagglutination). Interestingly the labelling alone did not seem to be the main reason because in some instances there was no decline in titer. The fractionation procedures used for preparing the globulins also caused a loss of antibody activity. Careful handling of the insulin antibodies during the labelling procedure as well as during the subsequent chromatography is necessary to obtain a good quality for immunohistological purposes. Furthermore the labelled antibody should be used immediately or kept at $-20°$; storage in the refrigerator led to a decline in titer within 3 days.

c) Immunofluorescence Studies of Various Organs

Investigation of the localization of antibody formation has shown that, according to the molecular size of the antigen, the capacity of aggregation of molecules and the techniques of detecting the antigen, the organs involved in the immunologic system exhibit marked differences. To our knowledge no exact observations relative to this question have been published for insulin, other than the preliminary work of PARKER, ELEVITCH and GRODKSY (1963).

α) Local Granulomatous Tissue

Incubation with FITC antibody: This involves either a globulin fraction obtained by $(NH_4)_2SO_4$ precipitation or a 7 S antibody obtained through the DEAE Sephadex A-50 column; both have total ability to bind insulin in pancreatic tissue.

At the site of antigen injection no appreciable amount of stored insulin could be detected in or on the cells, neither during the first few days nor in the following weeks and months. Occasionally minimal traces were found of intra- or para-cellular fluorescent material.

Incubation with FITC insulin: After the first two insulin injections no antigen-binding cells were observable. These cells appeared in the third week, lying individually in the thickly proliferated granulation tissue; some were typical plasma cells, and some histiocytes with a loose chromatin structure and cytoplasma. The number of these cells was low and remained constant during the following weeks and months. After the seventh month no antigen-binding cells whatsoever were detectable. The granulation tissue had progressed to fibrous, cell-poor scar tissue.

β) Regional Lymph Nodes

Incubation with FITC antibody: Neither at the beginning of the sensitization nor at a later point in time could an appreciable quantity of antigen be demonstrated in the lymph nodes under investigation (although in a few animals fluorescent material was present in the subcapsular and medullary sinuses).

Incubation with FITC insulin: Antigen-binding cells were observed for the first time 48 hours after the first injection of antigen. These lay singly in the medullary sinus and in the subcapsular sinus near the lymph follicles. These cells were relatively large with a large round nucleus and extensive cytoplasm, probably immature plasma cells; other cells were reticular types with branching cytoplasmic structure. In the following weeks the number of fluorescent cells increased continuously, though slowly. The predominant cells were mature plasma cells of type C (according to VASQUEZ, 1964). After the sixth week the number of fluorescent cells increased more definitely. With the mature plasma cells were large and medium sized lymphocytes, situated individually or in nests in the medulla and in the trabeculae.

Occasionally these cell nests were found within the germinal centers, although not often. The number of antibody-producing cells was greatest after 28 weeks (see Fig. 40) and again after further immunization at the 60th week. The antibody-producing cells lay in all parts of the lymph nodes, but principally in the transitional area from cortex to medulla.

A decline in antibody production was again seen in the regional lymph nodes of the two animals which had been immunized for a longer period of time (83 and 85 weeks respectively). There were essentially fewer cell nests present in cortex and medulla. Larger areas of the lymph nodes contained no such cells. A possible cause was the progressive cicatrization of the granulation area. The stimulus given by Freund's adjuvant was diminished compared with animals of a shorter immunization period.

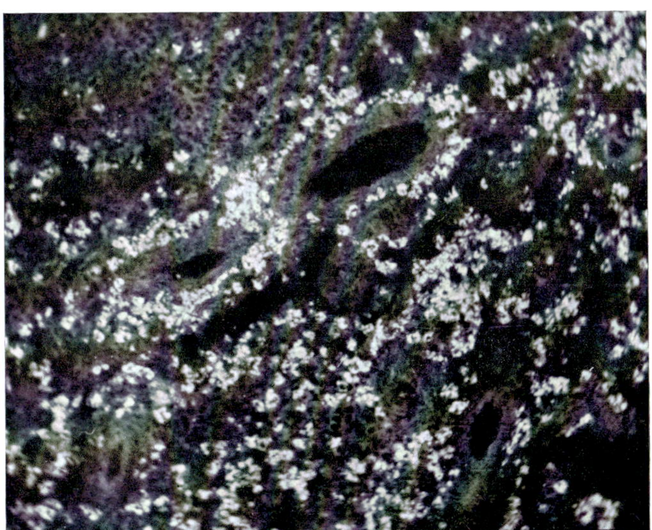

Fig. 40. Numerous antibody forming cells in a regional lymph node after 28 weeks of weekly immunization with insulin. Typical localization of antibody formation in the vicinity of vessels (periarteriolar lymph sheath). ×150

γ) Spleen

Incubation with FITC antibody: Until the third week no specific staining took place. Then in the following weeks occasional fluorescent cells were seen in the white and red pulp. These were large nucleated forms with branching cytoplasmic elements, probably macrophages.

Incubation with FITC insulin: In contrast to the regional lymph nodes, the spleen after only 24 hours evidenced lymphoid cells with relatively large nuclei and small cytoplasm in the periarteriolar lymph cell sheath at the rim of the red pulp (immature plasma cells). After the fourth day these cells were also found within the germinal centers. The number of these antibody-producing cells, which were diffusely scattered throughout, increased appreciably after the fourth week (Fig. 41 a). They occurred predominantly in nests in the red pulp (Fig. 41 b) and occasionally within the germinal centers.

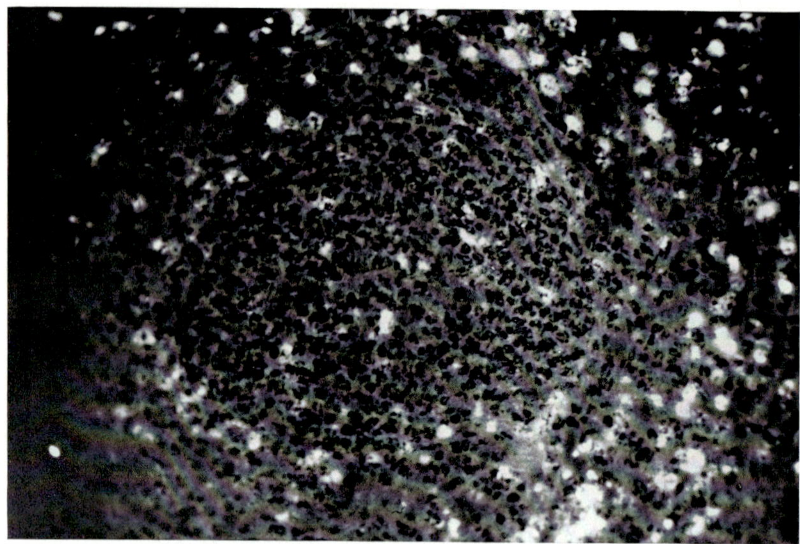

Fig. 41 a. Antibody-forming cells in the red pulp at the periphery of a Malpighian corpuscle. Scattered fluorescent-staining cells in the center. After 3 weeks immunization with insulin in guinea pig. ×180

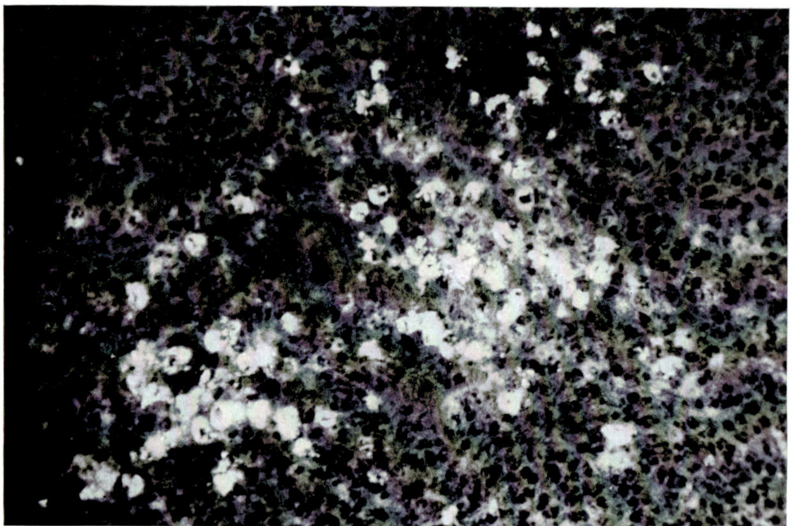

Fig. 41 b. Typical perivascular organization of antibody-forming cells in the spleen of guinea pig after 8 weeks' immunization. ×180

The perivascular regions were preferentially involved. In order to determine which cell types were active in antibody production, imprint preparations were made. Spleen cell imprints from normal control animals showed no uptake of FITC-insulin (Fig. 42).

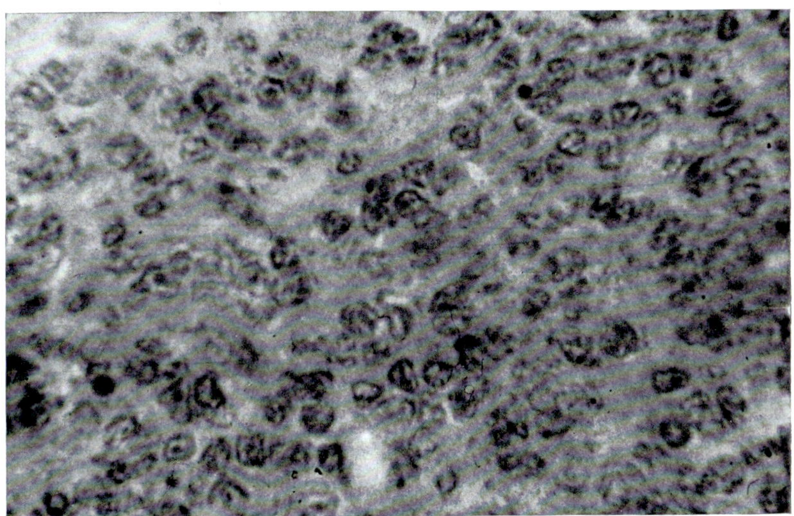

Fig. 42. Imprint preparation of the spleen of a control animal (guinea pig) after incubation with FITC-insulin. No specific fluorescence. ×480

The primary reaction against insulin appears to involve mainly large-nucleated cells with a small clear cytoplasmic ring-hemocytoblasts, or plasma cells of type A and B, according to VASQUEZ (1961). On the 5th and 6th days after the first administration of insulin mature plasma cells are seen (type C according to VASQUEZ) with a small nucleus, large cytoplasm and sometimes perinuclear clearing (Golgi apparatus, presumably).

In the course of further investigations, type B and C cells predominate, since the animals were always bled on the fourth day after the injection. Only in one animal immunized for a far longer time, which then died 12 hours after the last injection, did the immature cell forms again predominate. Differential counting in this animal resulted in: Type A 31% (Fig. 43 a); Type B 56% (Fig. 43 b); Type C 7% (Fig. 43 c); so-called lymphokinocytes (cells of lymphocyte size

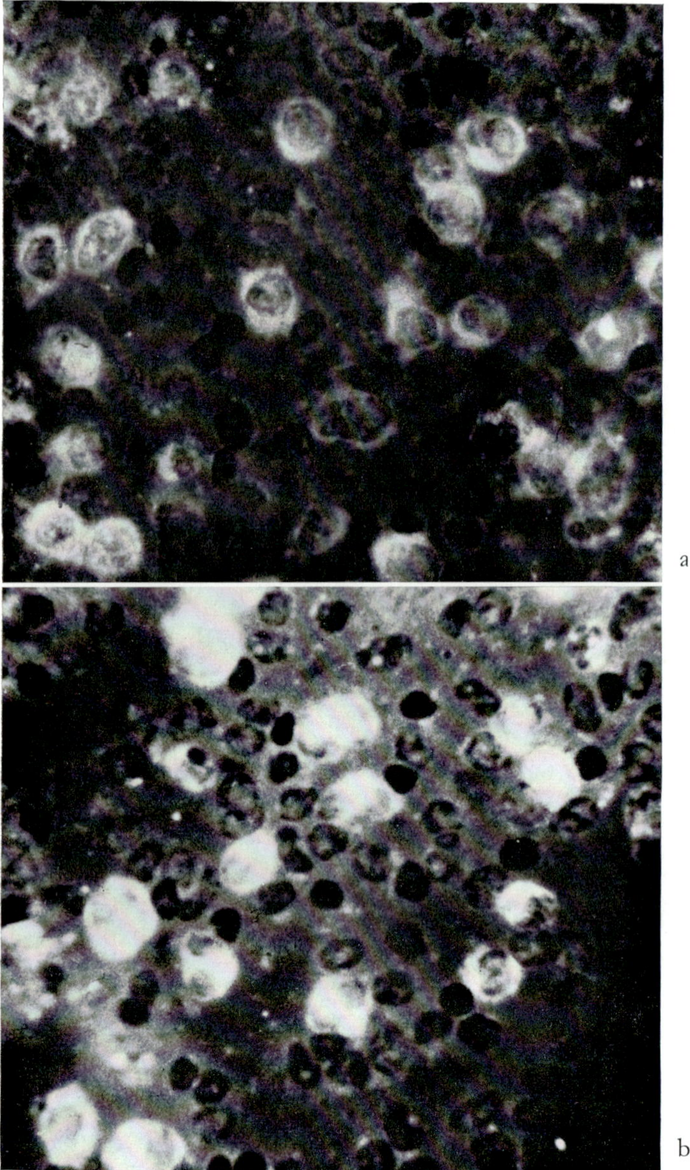

Fig. 43 a—b. Imprint preparations of the spleen of guinea pig no. 34 performed 12 hours after the last insulin immunization. Incubation with FITC-insulin after fixation with 95% ethanol. a Immature plasma cells of type A; b Immature plasma cells of type B (according to VAZQUEZ, 1964)

with a small fluorescing cytoplasm) according to VASQUEZ (1964): 6%.

The animal MS 31, which had also been immunized over a long period (85 weeks), was killed 4 days after the last administration of insulin, and exhibited the following differentiation of antibody-producing cells: Type A 2%; Type B 11%; Type C 83%; lymphokinocyte 4%.

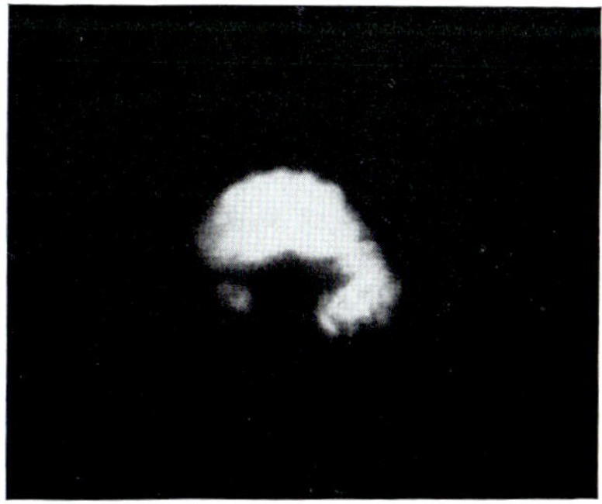

Fig. 43 c. Mature plasma cell type C according to VAZQUEZ (1964) from the spleen of guinea pig no. 31 4 days after the last immunization with insulin. ×1550

The number of antibody-producing cells in the spleen of these two longest-immunized animals was less than that of animals immunized for a shorter time. The titer of humoral antibodies was lower as well.

δ) *Bone Marrow*

An assessment of antibody-production in the bone marrow (femur) was possible only to a limited extent. The increased non-specific staining of the various cell types by both FITC antibody and FITC insulin allowed no more than the presumption that no appreciable antibody production took place here. Typical antibody-forming cells were found singly. Thus no demarcated cell populations (so-called "clusters") were recognizable, as had so clearly manifested antibody formation in the spleen and lymph nodes. The size and arrangement of these cells did not differ from that of the healthy control animals, which also showed quite intense non-specific staining.

ε) Liver

Incubation with FITC antibody: At no time in the sensitization could antigen be demonstrated in the liver.

Incubation with FITC insulin: During the first two weeks no antigen-binding cells were detectable. After the third injection there appeared diffusely scattered fluorescing cells. According to their localization, these cells were most likely Kupffer cells. Their number increased in the following weeks and reached its maximum after 28 weeks. In the animals immunized for longer than this, this type of fluorescing cell disappeared.

These cells lay along the sinusoids and displayed a large irregularly defined cytoplasm without a recognizable nuclear structure. The antigen-binding cells always occurred individually and never in the form of nests as in the spleen or lymph nodes. Cells resembling plasma cells were absent. Most probably these immunofluorescent findings indicate not antibody-formation, but rather antigen-binding by active RES-cells. A similar but less marked finding was observed in control animals which had at one time been immunized with Freund's adjuvant.

Summarizing then, continued immunization of guinea pigs against insulin manifests antibody production in the lymph nodes and spleen, while the granulation tissue and bone marrow play a subordinate role. No appreciable antibody-production occurs in the liver.

ζ) Kidney

With FITC antibody and FITC insulin no specific fluorescence could be detected in the areas of the glomeruli or tubules. This was equally true for the early days of immunization and for the later stages (maximum 85 weeks).

η) Pancreas

Incubation with FITC antibody: In the pancreas of all the experimental animals, with the exception of MS 34, mentioned above, the beta cells of the islets of Langerhans could be specifically demonstrated as in the control animals.

Incubation with FITC insulin: At no time in the immunization did a staining of the structures of the endocrine (Langerhans islets) or the exocrine pancreas occur.

Unprocessed cryostat sections: Unprocessed cryostat sections of the pancreas of all experimental animals exhibited no appreciable autofluorescence, with the exception of MS 34 which had been immunized for a period of 83 weeks with insulin. The islets of Langerhans demonstrated a pronounced yellow-green autofluorescence (Fig. 44)

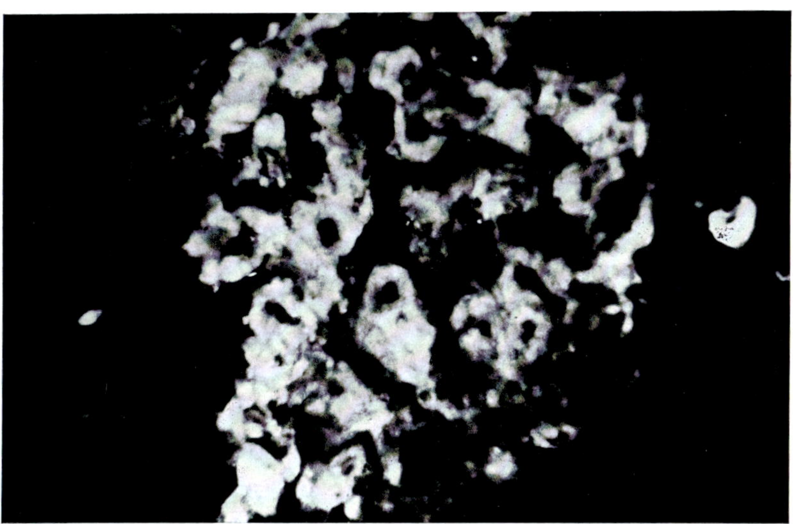

Fig. 44. Intense autofluorescence of a hyalinized islet of animal no. 34 (83 weeks immunization with insulin). ×480

which was not altered by treating the tissue. In the paraffin section (HE-stain) one could attribute the fluorescent appearance to a band-like hyalinized border of the islet tissues (Fig. 45 a, b).

Whether these structures were capable of binding FITC antibody or FITC antigen could not be determined owing to the intense autofluorescence.

d) Histological Studies

Routine histological investigations were performed on all the embedded renal and pancreas tissue of all experimental and control animals.

The study of the kidneys posed the question whether glomerular damage, in the sense of glomerulosclerosis (Kimmelstiel-Wilson,

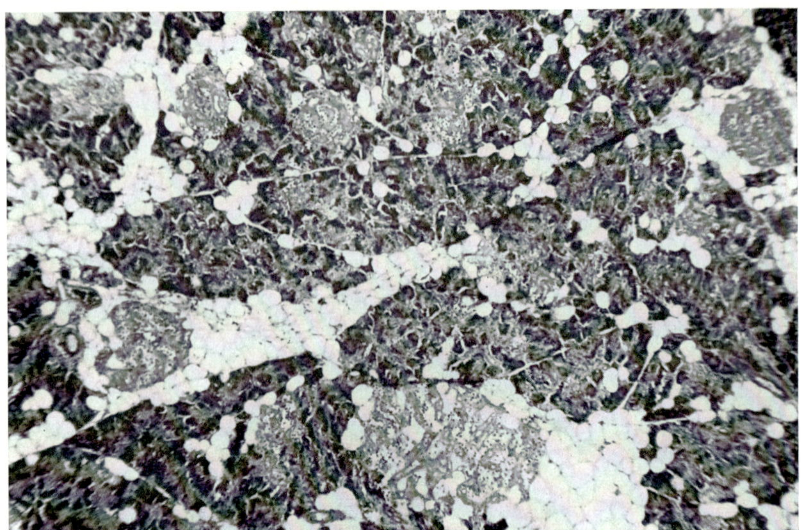

Fig. 45 a. Enlargement and hyalinization of the islets of Langerhans in animal no. 34 (83 weeks immunization with insulin). HE staining. ×120

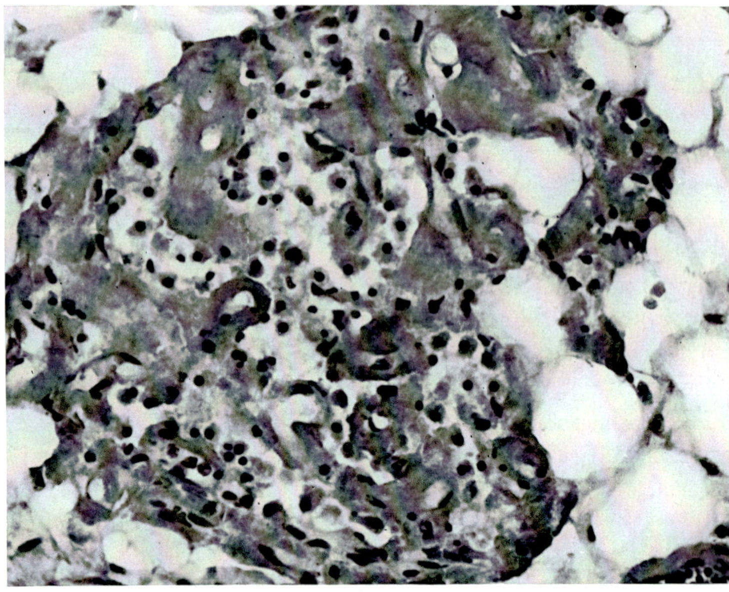

Fig. 45 b. Almost completely hyalinized islet of animal no. 34 with higher magnification. Endocrine cells no longer differentiable. The dark-staining nuclei with eosinophilic cytoplasm resemble the cellular findings in diabetic patients. HE staining. ×480

1936), could occur in the course of immunization to insulin, and whether the glomerular deposits detectable by immunfluorescence corresponded to this pathologic process. The study of the pancreas was expected to reveal whether alternatives to the islets of Langerhans do occur.

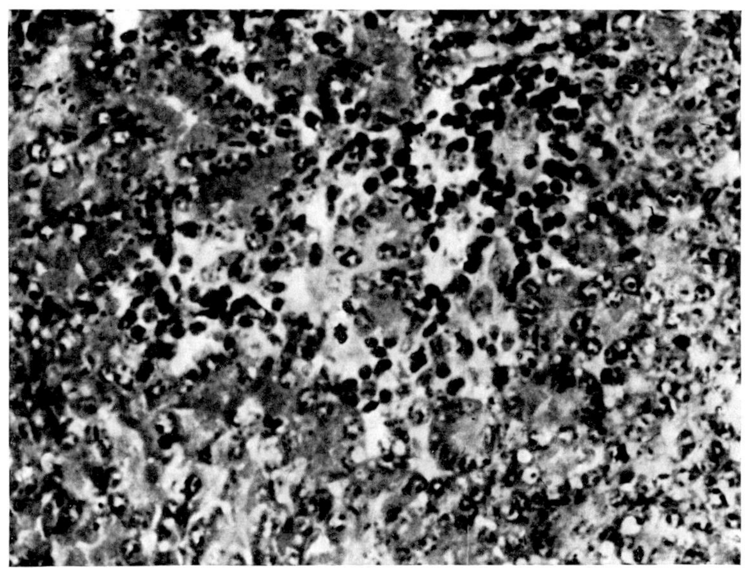

Fig. 46. Mild insulitis in a guinea pig after 8 weeks immunization with insulin. Infiltration of a small islet with mononuclear cells. HE staining. ×200

In none of the experimental or control animals were nodular glomerulosclerotic changes in the sense of Kimmelstiel-Wilson detected. Irregularly distributed thickening of the mesoangium and the basement membrane were found randomly.

The investigations of the pancreas evidenced in general no pathologic changes. The aldehyde fuchsin staining revealed A and B cells in normal number and size.

There were abnormal findings in two animals: animal MS 43, which had been immunized with insulin for an 8-week period, showed a small but significant infiltration of the smaller islets of Langerhans by mononuclear cells (Fig. 46), with suppression (replacement?) of the A and B cells, but without demonstrable necrosis. There also occurred in this animal a vessel wall swelling (to the extent of loss of lumen) in numerous islets.

Considerable pathologic changes were found in animal 34. The pancreas was already macroscopically enlarged. The essential finding was the enlargement and proliferation of Langerhans' islets. These islets demonstrated in part slight autolytic changes and desquamation of the A and B cells. The other islets were transformed into a hyaline mass (Fig. 45 a, b). Staining with Congo red for amyloid was negative. Inflammatory changes were absent.

3. Discussion

For clarity, the results of the various investigations will be discussed within certain frames of reference.

a) Blood Cells Producing Antibodies to Insulin

The investigations have shown that the technique of Cunningham is very suitable for demonstrating single cells producing anti-insulin antibodies. The number of lysed erythrocytes, which determines the extent of the diameter of the plaques (about 30—40 μ), corresponds to the results which Cunningham (1965) had obtained by coating erythrocytes with lipopolysaccharide of *Salmonella*. These results further demonstrate the same rhythm as other observers have reported in the appearance of circulating, antibody-producing cells. Thus Kearney and Halliday (1964) and Sorkin and Landy (1965) found the maximum number of antibody-forming cells in the circulation on the fourth day after the first antigen administration, followed by a decline to zero by the seventh day. The same authors noted an earlier peak in the antibody-producing cells, appearing on the third day after the second immunization. Kearney and Halliday, whose investigations were carried out in a similar way to our own, also observed a further decline in antibody-producing cells in the following weeks.

The cause of the occasional formation of plaques (circa 2/100,000) in control animals may well be a natural guinea pig antibody against rabbit erythrocytes. In the earlier reports of Jerne, Nordin and Henry (1963) the occurrence of random plaques in the vicinity of splenic cells of control animals was recorded.

The numbers of antibody-producing cells in the peripheral blood of the guinea pig given in these results are probably lower than the actual number present. Given the concept that not only true plaque formation but also the adherence and agglutination of erythrocytes to lymphoid cells could be an expression of their antibody activity — as CUNNINGHAM, SMITH and MERCER (1966) maintain — the same could apply to the present studies. Adherence to lymphoid cells and localized agglutination was observed but not quantitatively estimated. The number of antibody secreting cells is also expressed in these data. The antibodies released from the cells are most likely 19 S types; this type of antibody possesses a greater lytic activity in a complement-dependent system than do antibodies of the 7 S type. The latter form later and represent, so to speak, the mature humoral end product which is continuously synthesized as immunization continues. The present results reflect the following circumstance: after the first injection of insulin there is a latent period of 2—3 days, then a large number of antibody-producing cells are seen, declining as the interval after the administration of antigen lengthens. After the second injection, such cells appear sooner in the blood stream but there are fewer of them. As the titer of humoral antibodies climbs, these cells gradually disappear from the circulation. It seems almost certain that antibody synthesis is effected predominantly by the non-circulating cells of the immune system. Our technique was unable to indicate whether cells secreting antibody of the 7 S type were still circulating at this time. This sequence of events could be interpreted as follows: at the first exposure of the organism to the antigen, a flood of antibody-producing cells is released to achieve temporary neutralization at the site where the antigen is localized. This emergency mechanism ceases to function when the non-circulating lymphatic system is capable of producing adequate quantities of humoral antibodies.

b) Characteristics of the Humoral Insulin Antibodies in Guinea Pigs

Weekly injections, each of 20 units of insulin with CFA, induced the development of differing titers of antibodies in experimental animals, a phenomenon described in the early investigations of other authors. In most of the animals a "steady state" developed after 6 weeks. In only a few instances did the continued administration of antigen lead to much higher titers. The immunization procedure chosen was the regular administration of large amounts of insulin to simulate the situation of a diabetic patient; a different immunization regimen must be used to obtain the highest titers of antibodies. In agreement with MOLONEY and COVAL (1955), we found high titers when insulin was injected monthly (only two injections) and the animals were bled 14 days later. Antibody production, however, is also genetically dependent. WRIGHT and NORMAN (1966) divided guinea pigs into three types: antibody producers, nonproducers and latent producers. The last group began to produce active serum three months after they were first bled. Similar observations were made in our own investigations (Fig. 35). WRIGHT and NORMAN were able to convert nonproducers into producers by adding bacterial antigens (pertussis vaccine). Many other aspects (seasonal variations etc.) are of importance if the objective is to obtain active antisera but this is not the subject of this study. (For further information on this aspect, see HEINEMANN and FEDERLIN, 1971.)

Comparison between passive hemagglutination and ^{131}iodine binding of the antisera revealed no correlation in low titers while in higher dilutions the titers corresponded roughly. The reason for this finding is not clear. Possibly it depends on the type of antibody, because low titers in hemagglutination were mainly observed at the beginning of antibody production. A similar explanation was given by DECKERT (1964) for the different behaviour of rabbit insulin antibodies in passive hemagglutination and radioimmune electrophoresis. The capacity of antibodies to bind native insulin in tissue also corresponds roughly to the results of the hemagglutination test. A particularly good immunohistological demonstration of insulin in the beta cells of the rat pancreas is obtained with the highest antibody titers.

Several investigations have been carried out to characterize the types of antibodies to insulin which occur in guinea pigs. YAGI, MAIER and PRESSMAN (1962) found two different antibodies (beta and gamma region of globulins). In immunoelectrophoretic studies DECKERT (1964) demonstrated antibodies against pig insulin as gamma and beta 2 A globulins. HORINO, YU and BLUMENTHAL (1966) observed that most of the insulin antibodies contained two components one a slow moving gamma 1 globulin and the other faster migrating globulins (7 $S_{\gamma 1}$ and 7 $S_{\gamma 2}$). Surprisingly these authors also found in the first phase of immunization only occasionally 19 S antibodies; this may have been due to the schedule of immunization and sampling. Apart from this kind of characterization of insulin antibodies it is of interest to mention some other qualitative aspects. The antibodies directed against bovine insulin reacted not only with the antigen in soluble form, on the surface of erythrocytes, or in the tissue (bovine pancreas), but also with endogenous insulin of different species. MOLONEY and COVAL (1955) had shown for the first time an acute transient diabetes in mice after repeated intravenous injection of anti-bovine insulin antibodies from the guinea pig. WRIGHT (1959) established this finding in rabbits. KITAGAWA et al. (1960 a, b) had the same experience in mice, ARMIN, GRANT and WRIGHT (1960) in rats, rabbits and cats, CUNNINGHAM, PATTERSON and WRIGHT (1963) in sheep and cattle and SCHÖFFLING (1966) in dogs.

Insulin antibodies from other species (horse, sheep or even man), employed instead of guinea pig antisera, were able to reverse the hypoglycemic effect of insulin injected simultaneously in mice. Alone, however, these antibodies did not produce hyperglycemia. They seemed unable to neutralize endogenous insulin (WRIGHT et al., 1962). This was considered to be the special property of guinea-pig antibodies to insulin: This view (ROBINSON and WRIGHT, 1961) was shaken by the findings of PATTERSON et al. (1964), who were able to induce hyperglycemia in rats and dogs by using chicken anti-insulin anti-serum. ARMIN et al. (1961) found in extensive investigations that after administration of guinea-pig antiserum the biologically active insulin had disappeared from the serum of animals in the hyperglycemic state, that a high concentration of antibody-bound insulin was circulating for several days afterwards, and that 30 minutes after the injection there occurred a degranulation of the B cells in the islets of Langerhans. A fall in the insulin content of the pancreas was detected by extraction studies (GREGOR et al., 1963). Similar morphological findings were established by VON WATTENWYL and BÜRGI (1964). LACY and WRIGHT (1965) recorded an exudative inflammation of the islets of Langerhans accompanied by hemorrhage, necrosis, and leukocytic infiltration (in part eosinophils) after the administration of large doses of guinea-pig antisera to rats.

The particular property of guinea-pig antibodies against the endogenous insulin of other species necessitated the study of this reaction in guinea pigs which had previously been actively or passively sensitized. ARMIN, GRANT and WRIGHT (1960) had already shown that the transmission of guinea-pig anti-insulin antibodies to other guinea pigs induced no hyperglycemia. A reaction with the endogenous guinea pig insulin must have taken place. MANN and SMITH (1963) were able to observe a decline in insulin-like activity up to 30 days after a single injection of antibodies. This was the single piece of evidence in favor of a reaction between antibodies directed against heterologous insulin and the autologous guinea-pig insulin.

Thus there emerges the singular fact that different species develop antibodies to insulin but remain normoglycemic. This applies to the guinea pig as well. Guinea-pig antibodies (and probably those from chickens as well) are capable of evoking an immunologic diabetes in other species. POPE (1966) presumed therefore that the circulating antigen-antibody complex retains its biologic activity and that the antibody is directed solely against the antigenic determinants of the insulin molecule, which itself is not involved in the biologic activity. Why the intravenous injection of guinea-pig antibodies into other guinea pigs has practically no effect upon the blood sugar was not explicable.

Could the guinea-pig antibodies, in contrast to those of other species, penetrate the B cells of the pancreas and there bind to the insulin? The intravenous administration of rabbit anti-insulin serum to chicken embryos probably demonstrated just this reaction (BLUMENTHAL, BERNS and BLUMENTHAL, 1964). The rabbit antibodies were demonstrable in vitro within the B cells of the pancreas. The inflammation of the islets of Langerhans evoked by the massive administration of guinea pig antibodies to rats (LACY and WRIGHT, 1965) indicates a reaction of the antibodies with the insulin in the B cells. The binding of guinea-pig antibodies to the insulin of different species could be directly shown by means of immunofluorescence (LACY and DAVIES, 1957; LACY, 1959). However, insulin was not demonstrable in the pancreas of guinea pigs. This may probably be explained by the above-mentioned concept of the uniqueness of the guinea-pig antibody. The present morphological findings argue that the situation in guinea pigs is not basically different from that of certain other animal species. Thus, in contrast to LACY and DAVIES (1957, 1959) and to LACY (1959), our experiments with FITC-labelled antiinsulin antibodies of the guinea pig have shown that insulin was clearly demonstrable in the B cells of the islets of Langerhans in the same species. To be sure, the presentation of the B cells was weaker than in the species whose insulin was employed (cattle, pigs). The comparatively better staining with rat insulin is easily explained because rat insulin is chemically much more closely related to bovine or porcine insulin than the insulin of guinea pigs, which differs in the position of 18 amino acids.

After sensitization against heterologous insulin, guinea pigs could also be made diabetic. SENIOW (1966) obtained hyperglycemia in guinea pigs accompanied by weight loss and hyalinization of the islets of Langerhans, as in human juvenile diabetics.

Our own experiments with long term immunization of guinea pigs with heterologous insulin (porcine) did not produce a true diabetic state. Only one animal showed changes in the islets, in the form of a mild insulitis after 8 weeks of immunization, while another animal after two years of weekly injections of insulin developed hyalinization of all islets. The sudden death of the animal prevented the planned glucose tests of blood and urine. Interestingly, the islets showed a greenish-yellow autofluorescence rather similar to the picture which is observed after incubation of tissues with FITC-labelled compounds. So it was impossible to examine the pancreatic tissue immunohistologically. Hyaline degeneration of the islets of Langerhans was described for the first time by OPIE (1900) and is one of the most characteristic findings in elderly diabetics (OGILVIE, 1964; GEPTS, 1965). Because control animals of the same age showed no such changes of the islets, we incline to attribute the hyaline degeneration to the long-term immunization and not to age. SCHWARTZ, KURUCZ and KURUCZ (1965) described autofluorescence within islets of senile and presenile persons, but staining for amyloid in the guinea pigs's tissue was negative. The finding therefore remains unclear.

Already some years ago the labelling of insulin with fluorescein isothiocyanate for immunohistologic studies gave a basis for the investigation of possible changes in the antigenic properties of the insulin molecule. Thus HALIKIS and ARQUILLA (1961), using the passive hemagglutination test, found that erythrocytes labelled with FITC-insulin agglutinated at higher antibody concentrations than erythrocytes labelled with insulin alone. BERNS, HIRATA and BLUMENTHAL (1962) and PARKER, ELEVITCH and GRODSKY (1963) found no appreciable limitation of the antigenicity of FITC-insulin; however, they used a smaller quantity of dye in their insulin labelling experiments. Later ARQUILLA, OOMS and FINN (1966) reported that, after purification by acrylamide gel electrophoresis, FITC-insulin manifested the same biologic and immunologic properties as unlabelled insulin. The insulin used in the present investigations, prepared by Dr. MAGER of Hoechst, evidenced no altered antigenic qualities in the passive hemagglutination test and was nearly identical biologically to the unlabelled hormone. In biological testing of rabbits, 24.5 units of FITC insulin corresconded to 27 units of unlabelled insulin. Only a weakly labelled insulin should be employed for immunologic investigations; we used a molar F/P ratio of 0.1—0.5 (in patients a lower F/P ratio was used = 0.07).

Other experiments were performed with FITC-labelled anti-insulin antibodies. Here too, any alteration in the immunological properties can be studied by means of the passive hemagglutination test. Other antibodies have been investigated with various modifications (see literature review by VON MAYERSBACH, 1966) since the initial work by COONS and KAPLAN (1950). A precipitation reaction has been the most frequently used method of investigation. The loss of antibody activity is said to be small if the labelling is performed "in the usual manner" (VON MAYERSBACH, 1966). MARSHALL, EVELAND and SMITH (1958) showed that the use of organic solvents, such as acetone, in labelling proteins led to a decline in the titer of the antibody, which was often considerable, while FOTHERGILL (1964 b) considered the loss of antibody activity due to careful use of acetone to be minimal. However, this is irrelevant in the present experiments where labelling with FITC takes place on celite 10%, i. e. on kieselgur-bound FITC. A decline in the antibody activity can occur not only in the labelling but also presumably in the purification methods (gel filtration to separate the unbound dye). Corresponding observations were made by VON MAYERSBACH and GROSSI (1963). When further separation of the labelled antibody fraction was performed, using DEAE-cellulose, a loss of activity of 42—60% was observed (MCDEVITT et al., 1963). The insulin antibody employed in the present studies, which had been purified of free dye in a Sephadex G-25 column and was fractionated by DEAE-Sephadex (other sera were treated with ammonium sulfate to precipitate the globulin fraction) frequently showed a loss of activity on testing by the hemagglutination method. A fall in titer of 2—3 values could be observed. The loss was less marked if DEAE-Sephadex was used compared with the precipitation of globulins by ammonium sulfate.

c) The Localization of Antigen and Antibody Formation

The fate of injected antigen has been described in numerous experiments by many authors. COONS, LEDUC and KAPLAN (1951) were the first to describe the uptake of egg albumin, bovine albumin and human gamma globulin by the macrophages of the reticuloendothelial system (e. g. the spleen: sinus macrophages and the reticular cells of the red pulp) after intravenous injection in mice. In general these antigens were not demonstrable after a few days. Soluble protein antigens which were injected subcutaneously were found in the regional lymph nodes, or at the site of inoculation if Freund's adjuvant had caused granulation tissue to develop there. An antigen of small molecular size, such as insulin, which also possesses a high degree of metabolic activity, could not easily be demonstrated, as would have been expected. The rapidity with which the injected insulin was absorbed, despite emulsion with Freund's adjuvant, was apparent from the hypoglycemic shock occuring a few hours after the first injection. The fact that hypoglycemia did not occur with subsequent injections is more likely due to the rapid neutralization of the insulin by circulating antibodies than to an altered rapidity of absorption. It is not surprising that in the immunohistologic investigations of the injection site, i. e. in the local granulation tissue, only scattered traces of insulin are found in the macrophages. The regional lymph nodes contain scattered traces in the subcapsular and medullary sinus macrophages where the antigen was demonstrable by means of a labelled antibody. After the third week antigen-containing macrophages were detectable in the red pulp of the spleen and occasionally in the germinal centers (primary follicles). The development of antibodies to insulin was even more clearly demonstrated in the lymphatic antibody-synthesizing regions. It was stated above that the "sandwich" technique, utilized by WHITE (1963) and by VASQUEZ (1961, 1964) for the demonstration of antibodies against other antigens, yielded unsatisfactory results in the present investigations. The layering with unlabelled antigen and subsequent incubation with an FITC-labelled antibody against insulin brought either quite weak fluorescence of the those cells presumably containing antibodies, or no evidence at all of a specific reaction.

In contrast, the use of labelled antigen gave excellent results. Exactly the same observation was made by PARKER, ELEVITCH and

GRODSKY (1963) in their investigations of the localization of the formation of antibodies to insulin after short-term immunization. They suggested that this phenomenon occurs because the insulin molecule, which is poor in immunologically reactive groups, is capable of binding only upon one side. Our results with human leukocytes confirm this suggestion. The binding of antigen by sensitized cells with immunofluorescence was only possible by the direct method using labelled antigen. The antibody forming cells appeared in the regional lymph nodes and in the spleen, as with other antigens (COONS, LEDUC and CONOLLY, 1955; LEDUC, COONS and CONOLLY, 1955; ORTEGA and MELLORS, 1957; VASQUEZ, 1961, 1964; WHITE, 1963; FITCH and WISSLER, 1965). Remarkable was the occasional discovery of the first antibody-forming cells in the spleen just 24 hours after the subcutaneous injection of antigen — sometimes in combination with Freund's adjuvant. With this means of administration of the antigen, these cells might have been expected to appear after 3—4 days, although earlier after intravenous injection. The rapid absorption of insulin, even after subcutaneous injection, apparently induces an unexpectedly early appearance in the spleen. In general the localization of the antibody-producing cells corresponds to that described with other antigens, i. e. in the regional lymph nodes and in the spleen the cells were detectable in the subcapsular and medullary sinuses and as individual relatively large fluorescing cells in the red pulp. The primary reaction of the 3rd—4th day was somewhat weaker by the 6th day. The secondary reaction after the second subsequent injections is evidence of multiplication of the antibody-producing cells in the regional lymph nodes as well as in the spleen, although not in the granulation tissue. ASKONAS and WHITE (1956) also detected only very limited local production of antibody at the site of injection of antigen, even when the injection contained the adjuvant mixture of tuberculin bacilli. The antibody production is in this case more intense in the distant lymph nodes and in the spleen. But the use of incomplete Freund's adjuvant or aluminum phosphate precipitate gives abundant antibody-producing cells in the local granulation tissue. The injection site also determines the involvement of the regional lymph nodes in the antibody synthesis. For example, the use of the sole of the foot limited the protracted liberation of antigen to the proximal lymph nodes. Like PARKER, ELEVITCH and GRODSKY (1963), we chose the interscapular fad pad of the guinea pig as the site of injection in our investigations because this region has the advantage of allowing larger amounts of antigen adjuvant mixture to be injected as a depot dose. While the quantity of antibody-producing cells in the spleen continued to increase in the early weeks, reaching a maximum after 28 weeks and then declining (in the 83rd and 85th week in the hyperimmunized animals), an appreciable formation of antibody in the regional lymph nodes was observed in only two animals (28th and 60th weeks).

d) The Kidney in Long-term Immunization with Insulin

The nearly negative results of the histological and immunofluorescent studies of renal tissue in the long-term immunized guinea pigs are at variance with some observations of other authors. GRIEBLE (1960) found nodular hyaline glomerular lesions in rabbits treated for 24 weeks with long-acting insulin and human serum. The group of animals which received insulin alone showed no lesions comparable to the KIMMELSTIEL-WILSON changes in human diabetics. MOHOS et al. (1963) reported nodular renal lesions in only one rabbit after 6—7 weeks' immunization with heterologous insulin and complete Freund's adjuvant. In other animals they observed diffuse PAS-positive thickening of the basal membrane, arteriolar sclerosis with endothelial proliferation and inflammation of the interstitial tissue. BLUMENTHAL, GOLDENBERG and BERNS (1965) produced similar kidney lesions in rabbits after the same treatment and found fixation of FITC-insulin by the diseased glomeruli.

Of major interest to us are the experiments of MANCINI et al. (1969), also performed in guinea pigs. After 3—5 months of monthly injections of heterologous insulin plus incomplete Freund's adjuvant, they found PAS-positive hyaline nodules (55.5%), thickening of the basal membrane (100%), aneurysmatic dilatation of the capillaries (88.8%), diffuse glomerulosclerosis (61.8%), an increased number of mesangial cells (38.8%), fibrinoid caps (44.4%), and capsular adhesions (33.3%). Immunofluorescent studies of the lyophilized kidney sections showed staining of both the fibrinoid caps and hyaline nodules of the glomeruli with FITC-anti-insulin serum. The basement membrane and the intercapillary stroma (mesangial space) showed less fluorescence. The authors discuss three possible mechanisms underlying the renal lesions:

1. formation of tissue antibodies against insulin (MOHOS et al., 1963),

2. production of circulating anti-insulin antibodies which bind the insulin fixed to the glomerular basal membrane (GRIEBLE, 1960),
3. intracapillary binding of the antigen to the specific antibodies and production of a damaging immune complex (MOVAT, 1962).

However, the immunization of guinea pigs does not inevitably lead to such renal lesions, as our own experiments show, also the studies of FREYTAG and MENKE (1970) who similarly failed to produce glomerulosclerosis after immunization with heterologous insulin for several months. WEHNER, SCHADE and ASANTE (1969) observed "humps" on the outside of the loops in guinea pigs immunized with heterologous insulin. These authors interpret their findings as antigen-antibody complexes. They failed to find typical nodular lesions. The reason for such a different outcome of similar experiments in the same species may lie in genetic variations of the strains used, also in different modes of immunization.

A similar situation is seen in human diabetics who also do not inevitably develop glomerulosclerosis, even in long term insulin therapy. Because the theory of immune complexes postulates that living organisms can be divided into strong and weak antibody producers, it may be supposed that typical glomerulosclerosis occurs only in individuals who belong to the latter group, i. e. form complexes in antigen excess. These complexes are removed rather slowly from the circulation and can be fixed within the glomerular capillaries, presumably as a consequence of the anatomical arrangement of the renal circulation (HUMPHREY and WHITE, 1970). In this site they can cause an inflammatory response. In rabbits it was found that the best condition for producing glomerular lesions is to give a slight excess of antigen. This situation may exist in a certain number of diabetics and presumably experimental animals too.

4. Summary

Subcutaneous injection of 400 μg insulin (+ CFA) was able to produce the state of delayed hypersensitivity in guinea pigs. Fourteen days after sensitization, the skin test demonstrated a typical delayed type reaction. The existence of sensitized lymphocytes as carriers of the delayed immune reaction was shown by the migration inhibition test. These method was also used to investigate the antigenic elements of the insulin molecule, and it was shown that sensitized cells react not only with the complete insulin molecule but also with the polymolecular proinsulin and with (submolecular) isolated B chains. Reaction with the isolated A chain was so limited as to be statistically insignificant. Guinea pigs of the strain Pirbright white demonstrated a reaction with a synthetic insulin fragment of the B chain corresponding to the sequence B 11—16. Animals of another guinea pig breed did not react to the isolated fragment after sensitization with insulin. The development of sensitized cells depends, at least to some extent, upon a genetic factor.

Further, we were able to demonstrate direct binding of the antigen onto the sensitized blood-lymphocytes, as observed in patients with a delayed insulin allergy. The reaction was demonstrable both by immunofluorescence and by immunocyto-adherence.

The investigations of humoral antibodies showed that circulating antibodies to insulin are present during the state of delayed allergy to insulin. Both immunological mechanisms of the organism can exist simultaneously. An indication was found for a more intimate connection: animals with a very positive delayed skin reaction developed higher antibody titers during continued immunization than animals with a weakly positive skin test. The correlation was significant.

Our investigations of the appearance of antibody-forming cells in the blood after insulin sensitization utilized principally Cunningham's plaque technique. Here we demonstrated antibody-liberating cells from the circulation only a few days after the first injection of antigen. Their number declined in the subsequent weeks. The increase of circulating antibodies in the serum paralleled the decrease of these cells in the blood.

Immunohistological investigations of the sites of antibody formation revealed that the spleen is the organ in which the greatest number of antibody-forming cells were to be found. The local lymph nodes were the next most active organs. The local granulation tissue played an insignificant role in antibody formation. Further studies on the effect of long-term immunization (maximum 85 weeks) upon the kidneys and the pancreas indicated no real changes, such as glomerulosclerosis. Except in two animals, no changes were seen in the islets of Langerhans. In one animal complete hyalinization of the B cells was found; the etiology of this process could not be explained. Another animal demonstrated a slight infiltration of lymphocytes among the B cells (insulitis).

E. Appendix: Studies of Insulin-immunized Sheep

This work is presented as an appendix since the author was concerned mainly in the immunological investigations of the blood cells and the histological and immunological study of the pancreas of the experimental animals. The immunization of the animals with insulin was carried on during a 2-year period under the guidance of Professor A. E. RENOLD, director of the Institute of Clinical Biochemistry of the University of Geneva, by Dr. A. GONET. The author is much indebted to Prof. RENOLD, for manifold support during the cooperation in this work. Some results have been published jointly (FEDERLIN, RENOLD and PFEIFFER) in 1968.

I. Statement of Purpose

By sensitizing cattle to heterologous and homologous insulin, RENOLD, SOELDNER and STEINKE (1964) clearly demonstrated not only the presence of antibodies against the insulin, but also, in an investigation of the pancreas of the immunized animals, inflammation of the islets of Langerhans (insulitis). These studies, which were begun in the U.S.A., were continued in Geneva using sheep. This animal species offers certain advantages for such experiments — ease of care, in obtaining blood, etc. The purely lymphocytic character of the bovine insulitis implies that this could well be an immune reaction of the delayed type (LECOMPTE et al., 1966). An intracutaneous test dose of insulin evoked an extensive delayed allergic reaction in a sheep sensitized against insulin almost 2 years previously. The glucose tolerance test had given no suspicion of a diabetic state. But the investigation of the humoral antibodies indicated that antibody formation was directed not only against heterologous insulin but also against homologous, i. e. sheep insulin as well. The following account of the serological, immunohistological and immunocytological investigations presents some conclusions regarding the participation of sensitized cells and/or humoral antibodies in the state of experimental insulitis.

II. Results

The data pertaining to the tests on blood cells, tissue and serum are summarized in Tables 8, 9 and in Figs. 47—52. These results indicate that, in contrast to the two control animals, the 3 sheep sensitized to insulin developed humoral antibodies. The two animals treated with heterologous insulin developed antibodies against porcine and sheep insulin. In one porcine insulin treated animal very high titers were found. Slightly different results were obtained using passive hemagglutination and the maximum insulin-binding capacity. The former test gave high titers against the administered porcine insulin, while the latter yielded higher antibody titers against sheep insulin (Fig. 47). For technical reasons the immunocytological tests on blood cells provided inconclusive evidence that the insulin-sensitized sheep, especially animal no. 803 contained circulating sensitized lymphocytes.

Table 8. *Synopsis of the results obtained with immunohistological and histological examinations in insulin-immunized sheep*

No. of animal	Antigen	Incubation of frozen pancreas with FITC-insulin	FITC-anti insulin ab	FITC-anti sheep gammaglob.	Histology of paraffin embedded pancreas aldehyde fuchsin staining
119	Sheep insulin +FA	∅	+++	∅	No inflammation, typical beta-granules
221	Pig insulin +FA	∅	∅	∅	Weak lymphocytic infiltration of a few islets, typical beta-granules
803	Pig insulin +FA	++ Staining of lymphoc.	(+)	∅	Severe insulitis, only a few beta cells with typical granules
168	FA alone	∅	+++	∅	No inflammation, typical beta-granules
198	FA alone	∅	∅	∅	No inflammation, typical beta granules

Table 9. *Synopsis of the results obtained with serological, radioimmunological and immunocytological methods in insulin-immunized sheep*

No. of animal	Antigen	Serum antibody to sheep insulin		Serum antibody to pig insulin		Immune cytology	
		HAG	IBC	HAG	IBC	binding of FITC-insulin	immune adherence
119	Sheep insulin +FA	1 : 90	25 U/L	1 : 90	25 U/L	(+)	(+)
221	Pig insulin +FA	1 : 30	50 U/L	1 : 30	50 U/L	—	—
803	Pig insulin +FA	1 : 7290	2500 U/L	1 : 65610	700 U/L	(+)	(+)
168	FA alone	⌀	⌀	⌀	⌀	⌀	—
198	FA alone	⌀	⌀	⌀	⌀	⌀	—

HAG = Passive hemagglutination.
IBC = Maximum insulin-binding capacity.
⌀ = Negative result.
— = Examination not performed.
(+) = Positive results, but not quantitatively measurable.

The state of delayed hypersensitivity to insulin in these sheep was, however, clearly demonstrated by the skin test (Renold, Gonet and Vecchio, 1969).

Interesting findings were obtained in the studies of the pancreas. One of the three sheep sensitized to insulin showed severe inflammation of the islets of Langerhans, another limited infiltration of round cells. The insulitis observed in animal 803 (Figs. 48 and 49) gave a pathological picture analogous to that described by Renold, Soeldner and Steinke (1964) in cattle. The tissue adjacent to the islets, as well as the islets of Langerhans themselves, were infiltrated with round cells whose population consisted primarily of lymphocytes and some monocytes. Polymorpho-nuclear leucocytes were absent. Occasional plasma cells were found. On the edge of the islets in par-

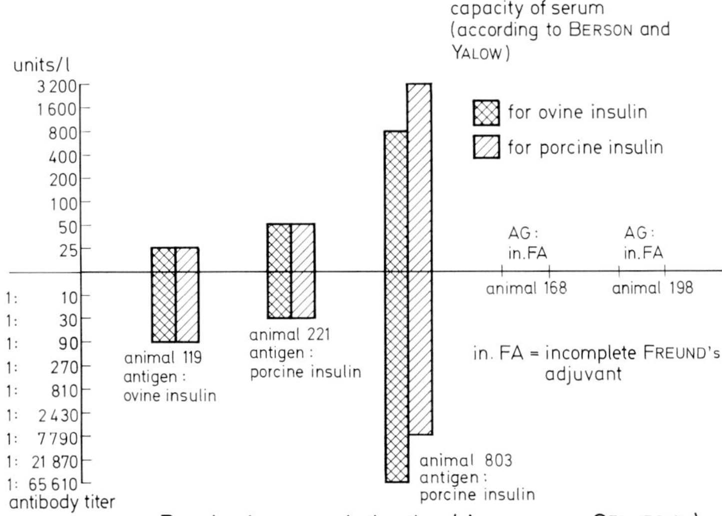

Fig. 47. Insulin antibodies in 3 sheep immunized with homologous (ovine) or heterologous (porcine) insulin plus incomplete Freund's adjuvant. Note cross reactions of antibodies with insulin which was not used for immunization

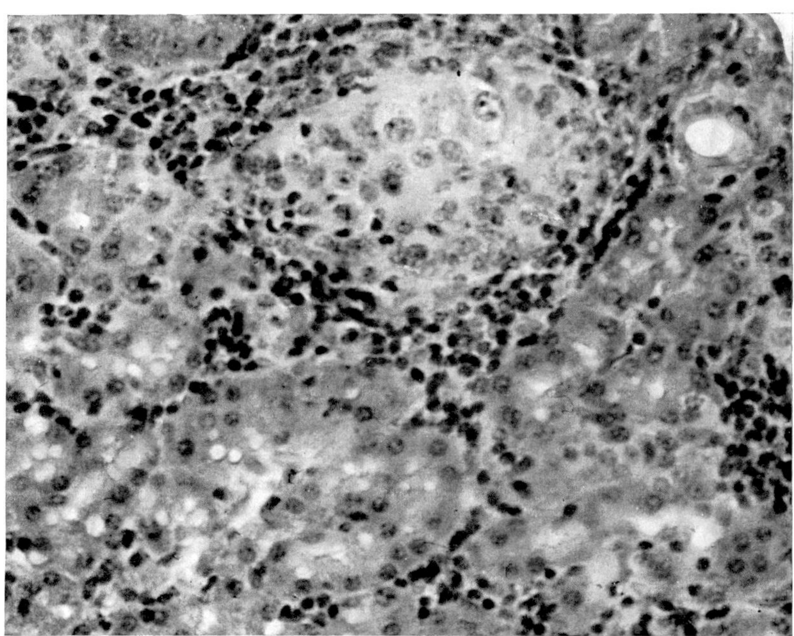

Fig. 48. Mild insulitis in sheep 803. Mainly periinsular collection of mononuclear cells. HE staining. ×200

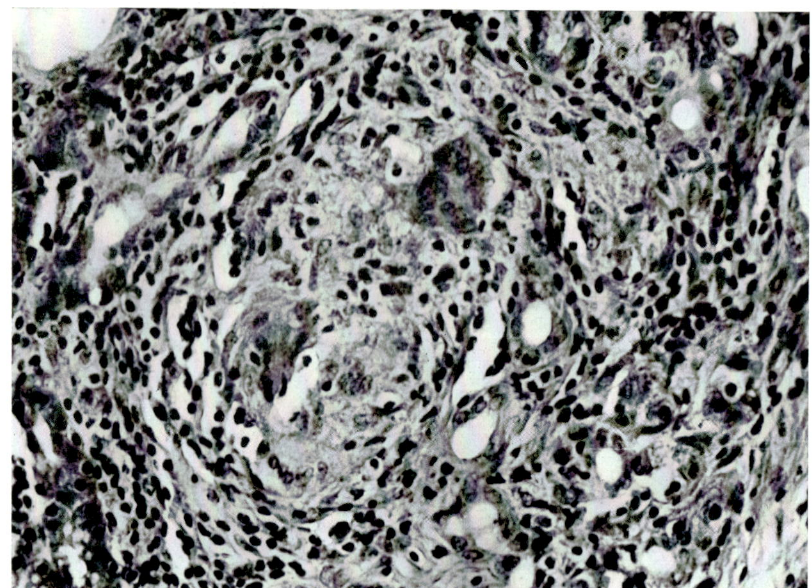

Fig. 49. Severe insulitis in sheep 803. Only a few remains of β-cells in the center of the islet. First signs of scarring in the surrounding tissue. HE staining. ×200

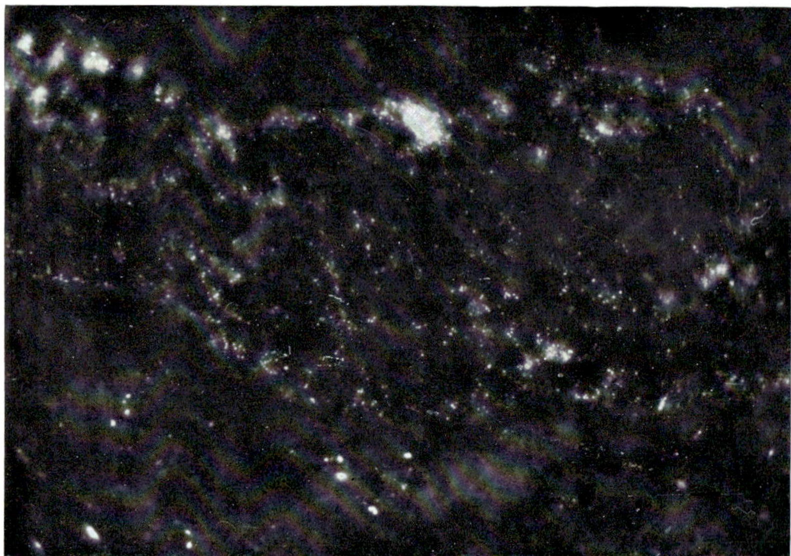

Fig. 50. Failure of demonstration of insulin by FITC-labelled antiporcine insulin-antibody of a guinea pig in sheep 803. Only a few scattered cells of the inflamed islet show reaction with the antibody. ×480

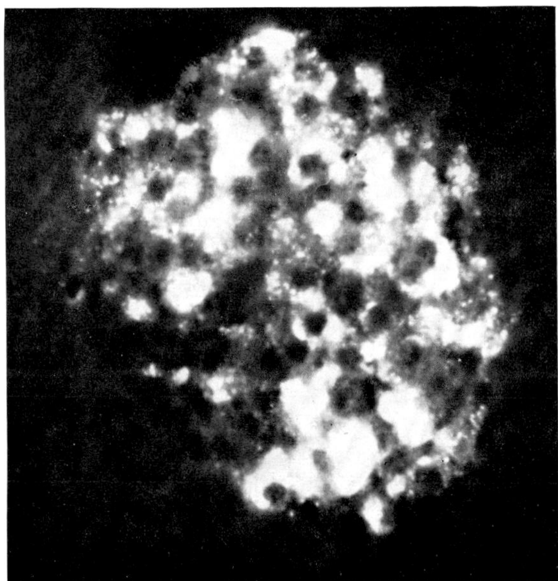

Fig. 51. Immunohistological demonstration of sheep insulin in a control animal with FITC-labelled anti-porcine insulin-antibody of a guinea pig. Cryostat section. ×480

Fig. 52. Some antigen-binding cells within the mononuclear infiltration of the islet tissue of animal no. 803. Incubation with FITC-insulin. Cryostat section. ×200

ticular partly loose and partly dense bundles of collagen could be distinguished. Within the inflammatory infiltrate the B cells were rarely of normal form, most being either pycnotic or greatly swollen. Staining with aldehyde fuchsin demonstrated the typical purple-colored granules in only a few fields. Similarly, the use of immunohistological techniques (FITC-labelled antibodies to insulin) revealed only traces of insulin within the islets in contrast to the immunohistological picture in sheep not sensitized against insulin (Figs. 50 and 51). Incubation with FITC-labelled insulin demonstrated the binding of this antigen to mononuclear cells within the inflammatory infiltrate (Fig. 52).

In the control sheep all serological and immunocytological investigations were negative, and the histologic evaluation of the pancreas revealed no pathologic changes in the islets; therefore no pathologic effect can be ascribed to Freund's adjuvant which has the effect primarily of intensifying the effect of the antigen.

III. Discussion

The observation in one of three sheep sensitized to insulin of a severe inflammatory reaction involving the islets, and in another animal of a mild inflammation, correlates with observations made in cattle and suggests a new aspect in the immunology of insulin. The organism, at least in these two species, not only develops humoral antibodies against the insulin administered, but attacks the sources of its own hormone as well, in the sense of an autoaggression. These observations from animal experiments would be of little moment — apart from their significance for experimental immunology — were it not for the fact that the pathology of humans offers an analogous example.

The term "insulitis" was originated by von MEYENBURG (1940) to describe the inflammatory infiltration of the islets of Langerhans in young diabetics, as mentioned initially by OPIE (1900) and extensively described by WARREN and ROOT (1925). Histologically the inflammation comprises principally lymphoid cells, some of which are small lymphocytes and some large round cells with a few polymorphonuclear granulocytes. Only rarely do the granulocytes dominate (WARREN and LECOMPTE, 1952). The inflammation is usually limited to the islets and involves alpha and beta cells equally in so far as both cell types are disturbed or replaced by inflammatory cells. In later stages the beta cells may be completely absent, while occasional alpha cells will be found. The islets themselves appear distorted and are often enmeshed in a network of edematous strands. A typical finding is the balling of the remaining islet cells into compact clusters (OGILVIE, 1964). The remaining endocrine cells possess a characteristically homogenous acidophilic cytoplasm and a very darkly stained nucleus. Abnormally large islet cells also occur which might be the morphological expression of a compensatory hypertrophy. Occasionally the inflammation extends into the adjacent exocrine portion of the pancreas.

Such an insulitis is seen only in a small group of diabetics, namely in children and adolescents, and then only if the diabetes is of short duration. Most observations have come from older reports since present progress in the therapy of diabetes enables most patients to survive their metabolic crises. Nevertheless up to the present insulitis is observed and described in the onset of diabetes (LECOMPTE, 1958; GEPTS, 1965, 1966). The bulk of diabetic patients exhibit no inflammatory changes, although this does not exclude their possible earlier occurrence.

The phenomenon of insulitis has been explained by various theories. Its frequent occurrence in children allows the assumption that the provocative agent could be a virus (SCHWARTSMAN, CRUSIUS and BEIRNE, 1947; JOHN, 1949; FARRELL, HAND and NEWCOMB, 1953; BROWN, 1956). Among other viruses, the mumps virus is particularly implicated, since there exist observations of the manifestation of diabetes in association with mumps (GUNDERSEN, 1927; COLE, 1934; KREMER, 1947; MELIN and URSING, 1958). It is worthy of mention that quite recently some pathologists have stated that they regard these changes as reactive (OGILVIE, 1964; GEPTS, 1966). From their standpoint a still unknown agent, of viral or bacterial nature, induces the degeneration of the islets and in some instances the hyperstimulation and subsequent death of the beta cells. The lymphocytic inflammation and the later connective-tissue proliferation are regarded as "reparative". LECOMPTE et al. (1966) state that a viral process is by no means incompatible with the findings. They cite the post-infection complications of many viral diseases which later continue as an autoimmune phenomenon, e. g. Hashimoto thyroiditis.

There is a strong histologic similarity between the picture described in human pathology and the insulitis produced in animal experiments (LeCompte et al., 1966; Toussaint and Gepts, 1966). But inferences to the pathogensis of insulitis in humans are possible at the present only in terms of scientific speculation in that a basic difference exists: humoral antibodies to insulin have not been definitely detected in untreated diabetic patients. New prospects are being opened up through modern insulin research, particularly the discovery of proinsulin. This was dealt with in Chapter B. V.

In the present studies an infectious agent was ruled out, spontaneously occurring insulitis being unknown in sheep, and finally Freund's adjuvant was not used in its complete form (dead tuberculosis bacteria), as this was certainly not an unimportant factor in other experiments on autoallergy; thus, there remains little to oppose the autoimmune theory as the explanation for experimental insulitis. The almost purely lymphocytic nature of the insulitis suggests the existence of a delayed type of hypersensitivity. This assumption would also apply to findings in cattle and in different immunopathologic state (Miescher, Dixon, Waksman cited by LeCompte et al., 1966). The results of the skin test, which are compatible with delayed hypersensitivity, further support this assumption. The morphological picture of the delayed hypersensitivity reaction was intensively investigated by Waksman (1960, 1962). The tissue changes which occur after contact with the respective antigen, whether they result from a skin test or from an experimental autoallergy with organ damage, conform to a fairly regular pattern:

1. Perivenous accumulation of mononuclear (sensitized) cells — predominantly lymphocytes and monocytes from the blood stream — immediately adjacent to the tissue containing the antigen.
2. Further increase of these cells by additional cells or by cell division.
3. Penetration by histiocytes into the antigen-containing organ.
4. Destruction of the antigen-containing elements by the histiocytes.

The culmination is loss of parenchyme, with or without evidence of regeneration, and with residual inflammatory cells and fibrosis. If these descriptions agreed with the findings in the pancreas, insulitis could be regarded as a typical example of experimental autoallergy. However, the pathogentic mechanisms are not well understood.

Whether sensitized cells or serum antibodies to antigen play the decisive role in the damage to the organ remains uncertain, despite the very exact experimental studies of autoallergic mechanisma in thyroiditis and encephalomyelitis. The theory of the so-called "combined reaction" (GELL and BENACERRAF, 1961) is advanced as an explanation for the synergistic action of sensitized cells and humoral antibodies. This possibility is lent credence by the fact that the animal (803) with the highest titer of serum antibodies to insulin experienced the most extensive pancreatic destruction. It remains difficult to understand that no gamma globulin was demonstrable by means of immunfluorescent examination of inflamed tissue. This finding was confirmed by CRUCHAUD (1966) in Geneva, in studies of the same sheep pancreas.

Regarding the question as to how contact occurs between sensitized cells or humoral antibodies and the antigen, RAFFEL (1965) proposed a choice of possible initial events:

1. The sensitized cells are drawn to the antigen by chemotaxis.

2. The sensitized cells penetrate the perimeter of an antigen-laden area by accident, and come into contact with antigen; an antigen-antibody reaction results, and develops into a mild inflammation which increases the local vascular permeability; among the now greatly increased cells are present many sensitized cells which react with the antigen and enhance the inflammatory process.

3. Small quantities of serum antibodies initiate the reaction in which certain pharmacologically active substances are liberated by binding to antigen, as in the immediate reaction. But because of the minute concentration of antibody present, it does not proceed to an actual immediate reaction. The reaction, however, does initiate vascular dilation and increased permeability of the vascular wall so that sensitized and non-sensitized cells can penetrate. The dominant process now becomes the reaction of cell-bound antibody with antigen. Since insulin is secreted into the blood stream, the binding of antigen to sensitized cells would be by the nature of the process quite possible. That the humoral antibodies can apparently arrive at and even penetrate the B cells is reported in the findings of BLUMENTHAL, BERNS and BLUMENTHAL (1964). These workers had found that a rabbit antibody to insulin could be found *within* the B cells of chick embryos after intravenous injection. Although this discussion is limited primarily to sensitized cells and humoral antibodies, it should

be emphasized that the other reagent, the antigen insulin, is full of uncertainties. It is by no means a uniform substance. The discovery of pro-insulin (STEINER, 1967) and of other components of insulin extracts (SCHLICHTKRULL et al., 1969) requires that the immunogenicity of these substances be investigated.

Finally, in order to permit a functional comparison to conditions in man, one must ask if experimentally-induced insulitis can lead to the state of diabetes. The studies by RENOLD of immunized cattle and sheep do not answer this question because the animals were killed at a time when the glucose metabolism was not altered by the already-present insulitis. Apparently the production of insulin by the functioning islets of Langerhans (even with the production of newly formed B cells) was adequate to meet the demands of glucose tolerance tests. Whether the insulin level in the serum was elevated, as in humans, before the manifestation of diabetes remains open to question. In another species the question of diabetes following insulitis has already been answered. TORESON et al. (1964) and GRODSKY et al. (1966) were able to induce insulitis with severe, lasting diabetes in rabbits sensitized to bovine insulin. Complete destruction of the B cells occurred. There is a distinct probability that these sensitized cattle and sheep might have developed diabetes given sufficiently long survival. The finding in rabbits confirms the well-known experience that for the induction of an experimental autoimmune illness it is immaterial whether heterologous or homologous tissue is employed as antigen. In general it is recognized that rabbits have a special position in this regard, as in this species the injection of foreign tissue leads to more intense development of autoantibodies than the injection of homologous tissue (WEIGLE, 1963; ASHERSON and DUMONDE, 1964). These few but significant findings for autoimmune diabetes in animal experiments again raise the question as to whether there exist parallels to (human) juvenile diabetes — apart from the morphologic correlation. The ability to demonstrate that a spontaneous autoimmune process is the cause of juvenile diabetes is lacking at present. Indeed, MANCINI, ZAMPA, VECCHI and ZAMPA (1965), found antibodies to insulin in untreated diabetics, by means of immunofluorescence; however these results have not so far been confirmed. But observations made more and more frequently in the last few years, that genuine autoimmune diseases arise spontaneously, e. g. thyroiditis (see the review by FEDERLIN, 1969), suggest that genetic alterations of the immune mechanism may permit spontaneous destructive processes in the islets themselves. However, this cannot be true for the majority of juvenile diabetics. There remains the hypothesis that an exogenous trigger (virus?) may make the B cell (or its content) susceptible to autoaggression.

The insulitis described above must not be confused with the so-called allergic interstitial pancreatitis induced experimentally in rats by i. p. or. i. r. injection of guinea-pig anti-insulin serum (LACY and WRIGHT, 1965; WRIGHT, 1969), which induces a transient diabetic state. In the majority of the animals in this model, eosinophilic leukocytes were seen to be infiltrating the acinar tissue of the exocrine gland as early as 4 hours after injection of the serum. In a smaller proportion of these animals, pancreatic edema and focal necrosis or hemorrhage affecting a few acini within the lobules was observed. The authors did not observe necrosis or hemorrhage of the islets of Langerhans, which showed only slight cellular infiltration and degranulation of the beta cells. Recently FREYTAG, MITSCHKE and KLÖPPEL (1970) reported species-differences in the histological response of the islets of rats and mice after i. r. administration of guinea pig anti-insulin serum. While rats developed a transient acute inflammation with emigration of polymorphonuclear and eosinophilic leucocytes, mice showed a chronic irreversible insulitis which was followed by persisting diabetes. Because this type of insulitis could be transferred to untreated mice by spleen cell, the authors suggest autoimmune mechanisms to be involved. A similar lesion (but without edema, hemorrhage and necrosis) is found in the pancreas of some infants born of insulin-treated diabetic mothers and dying a few days after birth, as described in detail by MCKAY, BENITSCHKE and CURTIS (1953), SILVERMANN (1963). In such cases the eosinophilic infiltration of the acinar tissue is accompanied by diffuse interstitial fibrosis. Because insulin antibodies may cross the placental barrier, it is not impossible that this human condition represents a form of pancreatitis very similar in etiology to the experimental model in rats.

IV. Summary

Three sheep were immunized subcutaneously at 14-day intervals with insulin and incomplete Freund's adjuvant over a period of almost 2 years. There were intervals of several weeks or even months when no injections were given. In two animals the antigen employed was porcine insulin, in the third ovine insulin. Two other sheep, acting as control animals over the same period of time, received only incomplete Freund's adjuvant.

The experimental animals developed humoral antibodies against both the foreign insulin and the species-specific insulin. Passive hemagglutination and maximum insulin-binding capacity of serum showed only little differences. In two animals there occurred only weak antibody formation, while in the third it was intense. The histological investigation of the pancreas in the third animal evidenced a striking infiltration of lymphocytes into the islets of Langerhans and adjacent areas, with diffuse depletion of the A and B cells. A few inflamed areas were found in one of the other two animals, while the fourth gave no indication of pathologic changes in the pancreas. The animal with marked insulitis gave a strongly positive delayed allergic reaction to the intracutaneous injection of insulin. This appeared to indicate the existence of sensitized lymphocytes. It was possible by the use of immunofluorescence to prove the binding of insulin by cells of the inflammatory area in the pancreas. There was no evidence of the involvement of humoral antibodies of the sheep.

The results indicate that together with the formation of antibody against exogenous pancreatic insulin there occur immune reactions with endogenous pancreatic insulin, which process can be designated as a form of autoaggression.

Note added in proof

Further studies in insulin-immunized rabbits support the hypothesis that sensitized lymphocytes play the dominant role in experimental insulitis. Lymphocytic infiltration of the islets occurred even before circulating antibodies to insulin were detectable. The lymphocytes were frequently observed in close contact with beta cells. With electron microscopy it was found that the lymphocytes inserted pseudopodes between islet cells which showed a reduction of secretion granules. (LEE, J. C., GRODSKY, G. M., CAPLAN, J., CRAW, L.: Experimental immune diabetes in the rabbit. Amer. J. Path. **57**, 597, 1969.)

F. General Summary

The investigations have been concerned with the various kinds of immune reactions, in man and in experimental animals, which follow the injection of insulin. Accordingly the immunogenicity of insulin was reviewed and the methods by which it had been investigated, the types and characteristics of the humoral antibodies and the hitherto sparse studies of the delayed immune reaction to insulin. To this section some general aspects of cell-mediated immunity were added. Furthermore, examples were given of the clinical symptoms of the various forms of insulin allergy and insulin resistance.

The delayed local allergic reaction following injection of insulin in diabetics is thoroughly discussed. To show that a cell-mediated immune reaction is, in fact, the mechanism involved, immunofluorescence and immune adherence were employed to demonstrate direct binding of antigen by the circulating white blood cells. The principles and technical details of immunofluorescence are discussed, including the labelling of insulin and insulin antibodies with fluorochrome and how this procedure influences the immunological and biological properties of insulin. These methods were applied to isolated blood cells and the evaluation of the preparations is described. Furthermore the lymphocyte transformation test was performed in patients with insulin allergy of the delayed type, and the serum was tested for the presence of humoral insulin antibodies, intracutaneous skin tests were performed with various types of insulin and finally, in some instances, skin biopsies were examined histologically. Fourteen patients with delayed allergy to insulin were investigated either at the beginning or at the end of the allergic symptoms. The skin reaction developed usually 10—12 hours after the injection of insulin, in some cases after 24 hours, receding in 2—3 days. Antigen binding by circulating lymphocytes was observed when the investigations were performed at the onset of the reaction. Antigen binding by granulocytes, too, was found during the later stages of insulin allergy. While the antigen-binding of the lymphocytes characterizes the delayed type of immune reaction, the detection of antigen-binding by granulocytes suggests—at our present state of knowledge—the involvement of humoral antibodies, secondarily absorbed into the blood cells. No patient with delayed allergy to insulin evidenced reagins in the serum. Neutralizing antibodies were already present at the time of the delayed allergic reaction. Tests of insulin binding in control subjects yielded a maximum of 6% positive leucocytes (mixed cells): the percentage in patients with delayed insulin allergy was clearly higher. From the technical standpoint, one might assume that the percentage of positive lymphocytes in vitro is higher than the effective number of circulating cells which are capable of binding antigen. In three patients with the signs of a delayed localized reaction to insulin, no significant antigen binding by circulating cells could be observed, but this may have been because only one examination of cells could be done (the patients did not return to the out-patient service for unknown reasons). In five patients a generalized reaction to insulin of the immediate type was observed. These patients did not demonstrate antigen binding by circulating blood cells. In two patients the demonstration of reagins in the serum (with the AST-test of LAYTON et al.) was performed.

Allergy and resistance to insulin can occur simultaneously or successively. The relationship between these two immune reactions is discussed.

The delayed allergy to insulin and the development of humoral antibodies were then investigated in experimental animals. A typical delayed reaction to insulin, fully analogous to the reaction observed in man, can be induced in guinea pigs with 400 μg insulin emulsified in complete Freund's adjuvant. This reaction could be transferred via the lymphocytes to normal animals. The migration inhibition test with peritoneal exudate cells of the sensitized animals was strongly positive. The reactivity of the sensitized lymphocytes involved not only the complete insulin molecule, but also the B-chain and, in one strain of guinea pigs, even a synthetic insulin fragment with the amino acid sequence B_{11-16}. The investigations of humoral antibodies clearly showed that their production has begun when the ability to evidence a delayed type reaction is present. The two immune systems have associations. Humoral antibodies react with both isolated chains.

During the state of delayed hypersensitivity antigen binding by peripheral lymphocytes was observed by means of FITC-insulin and insulin-coated erythrocytes (immunocytoadherence), although to a lesser degree than in humans.

At the beginning of immunization there are cells present in the peripheral blood which produce insulin antibodies and which disappear after the onset of the production of humoral antibodies within the sessile immune system, i. e. after the appearance of insulin antibodies in the circulation. By weekly subcutaneous administration of insulin with CFA an antibody peak was obtained after 4—6 weeks in the majority of the animals. In a few animals the titer increased with continuous immunization. However, when the antigen was administered at intervals of 4 weeks and the animals bled after 2 weeks, much higher titers were obtained. Titers were measured by passive hemagglutination and by binding of ^{131}iodine-labelled insulin. At low titers hemagglutination was less sensitive, but with increasing antibody titers a good correlation was shown between the two methods.

By means of FITC-labelled insulin antibodies, insulin could be demonstrated immunohistologically in the beta cells of various species. Cryostat preparations and freeze-dried material and preparations fixed in formaldehyde and imbedded in paraffin could be utilized, but other methods of fixation could not. Histologic and immunohistologic investigations of various organs were undertaken after long-term immunization (up to 85 weeks with weekly immunization). Antibody production occurred primarily in the local lymph nodes and in the spleen. The local granulomatous tissue was weakly involved in the antibody production. Despite the weekly injections of 20 units of insulin for many months, the animals developed no renal changes resembling Kimmelstiel-Wilson's glomerulosclerosis. One animal showed a mild insulitis after 8 weeks immunization, and another complete hyalinization of the islets of Langerhans after 85 weeks.

In the appendix, investigations are described which were performed in sheep at the Institut de Biochimie Clinique, Geneva, by Professor Renold and his colleagues: 3 animals were immunized with ovine or porcine insulin and incomplete Freund's adjuvant. They developed antibodies directed against both types of insulin, no matter which was used as antigen. A severe insulitis (autoimmune insulitis) occurred in one animal, a mild form in another. As with other autoimmune diseases, the immunologically competent cells seemed to be mainly responsible for the tissue damage. Its resemblance to insulitis in juvenile diabetics is discussed. — A schematic survey of the immune reactions to insulin is given in Fig. 53.

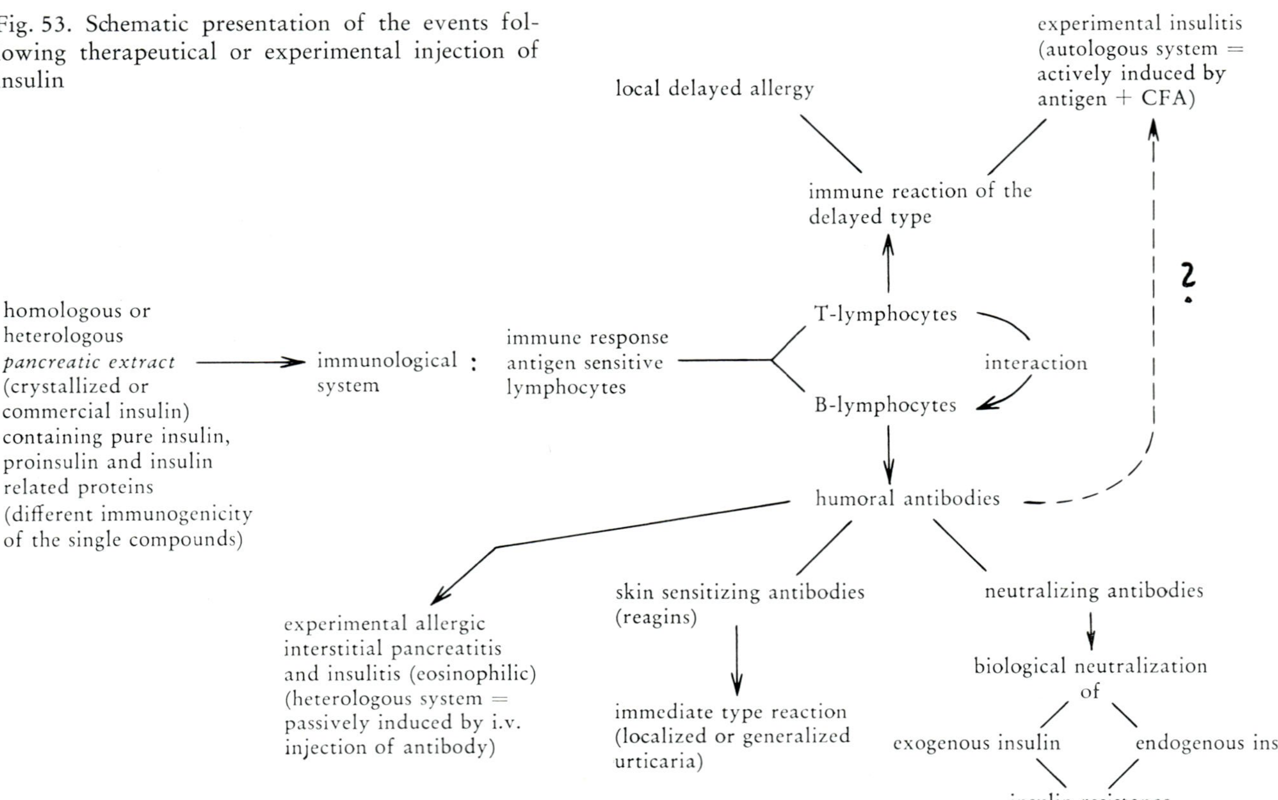

Fig. 53. Schematic presentation of the events following therapeutical or experimental injection of insulin

References

ADAM, W.: Insulin. In: Klinik und Therapie der Nebenwirkungen. Hrsg.: H. P. KUEMMERLE, A. SENN, P. RENTCHNICK u. N. GOOSSENS. Stuttgart: Georg Thieme 1960, S. 775.

ALLAN, F. N., SCHERER, L. R.: Insulin allergy. Endocrinology **16,** 417 (1932).

ANDREANI, G., CORTI, L.: Allergy to insulin: Statistical study of 1,500 diabetics. J. Amer. Med. Ass. **157,** 184 (1955).

ARKINS, J. A., ENGBRING, N. H., LENNON, E. J.: The incidence of skin reactivity to insulin in diabetic patients. J. Allergy **33,** 69 (1962).

ARMIN, J., GRANT, R. T., WRIGHT, P. H.: Acute insulin deficiency provoked by single injections of anti-insulin-serum. J. Physiol. (Lond.) **153,** 131 (1960).

— CUNNINGHAM, N. F., GRANT, R. T., LLOYD, M. K., WRIGHT, P. H.: Acute insulin deficiency provoked in the dog, pig and sheep by single injections of anti-insulin serum. J. Physiol. **157,** 64 (1961).

ARNON, R., SELA, M.: Studies on the chemical basis of the antigenicity of proteins. 2. Antigenic specificity of polytyrosyl gelatins. Biochem. J. **75,** 103 (1960).

ARQUILLA, E. R.: Relationships between A and B chain, necessary for antigenic determinants and the biologic activity of insulin. VIth Congr. Int. Diab. Fed. Stockholm, 1967. Ref. Abstr. diabetol. (NOVO) III, 134 (1967).

— BROMER, W. W., MERCOLA, D.: Immunology conformation and biological activity of insulin. Diabetes **18,** 193 (1969).

— OOMS, H., FINN, J.: Genetic differences of combining sites of insulin antibodies and importance of c-terminal portion of the A-chain to biological and immunological activity of insulin. Diabetologia **2,** 1 (1966).

— STAVITSKY, A. B.: The production and identification of antibodies to insulin and their use in assaying insulin. J. Clin. Invest. **35,** 458 (1956 a).

— — Evidence for the insulin specificity of rabbit anti-insulin serum. J. Clin. Invest. **35,** 467 (1956 b).

ARRHENIUS, S., MADSEN, TH.: Anwendung der physikalischen Chemie auf das Studium der Toxine und Antitoxine. Z. Phys. Chem. **44,** 7 (1903).

ARSDEL, P. P. VAN, SELLS, C. V.: Antigenic histamine release from passively sensitized human leukocytes. Science **141,** 1190 (1963).

ASHERSON, G. L., DUMONDE, D. C.: Autoantibody production in rabbits. V. Comparison of the autoantibody response after the injections of rat and rabbit liver and brain. Immunology **7,** 1 (1964).

ASKONAS, B. A., WHITE, R. G.: Sites of antibody production in the guinea pig. The relation between in vitro synthesis of antiovalbumin and gamma-globulin and distribution of antibody-containing plasma cells. Brit. J. exp. Path. **37,** 61 (1956).

BÄNDER, A.: Personal communication (1966).

BANTING, F. G., FRANK, W. R., GAIRNS, S.: Anti-insulinactivity of serum of insulin treated patients. Amer. J. Psychiat. **95,** 562 (1938).

BARTELHEIMER, H.: Insulinbedingte Hautnekrosen bei einem Diabetiker. Schweiz. med. Wschr. **82,** 573 (1952).

BAUER, J., KUNEWAELDER, E., SCHÄCHTER, F.: Über Antihormon. Wien. klin. Wschr. **50,** 83 (1937).

BEHRENS, O. K., BROMER, W. W.: Biochemistry of the protein hormones. Amer. Res. Biochem. **27,** 57 (1958).

BERNS, A. W., HIRATA, Y., BLUMENTHAL, E. T.: Application of fluorescence microscopy to the study of possible insulin binding reactions in formalinfixed material. J. Lab. Clin. Med. **60,** 535 (1962).

BERSON, S. A., YALOW, R. S.: Quantitative aspects of the reaction between insulin and insulin-binding antibody. J. Clin. Invest. **38,** 1996 (1959 a).

— — Species-specificity of human antibeef, -pork insulin serum. J. Clin. Invest. **38,** 2017 (1959 b).

— — Antigens in insulin. Determination of specificity of porcine insulin in man. Science **139,** 844 (1963).

— — Demidation of insulin during storage in frozen state. Diabetes **15,** 875 (1966).

— — BAUMANN, A., ROTSCHILD, M. A., NEWERLY, K.: Insulin-131-I metabolism in human subjects: Demonstration of insulin binding globulin in the circulation of insulin treated subjects. J. Clin. Invest. **35,** 170 (1956).

BIEDERMANN, M.: Untersuchungen über zirkulierende Zellen im Blut mit Antikörperbildung gegen Insulin. Thesis. University of Ulm, 1969.

BIRKENSHAW, V. J., RANDALL, S. S., RISDALL, P. C.: Formation of precipitin lines between insulin and anti-insulin serum produced in sheep and in guinea pigs. Nature **193,** 1089 (1962).

BLOOM, B. R., BENNETT, B.: Migration inhibitory factor associated with delayed hypersensitivity. Fed. Proc. **27,** 13 (1968).

BLUMENTHAL, D. D., BERNS, A. W., BLUMENTHAL, H. T.: Anti-insulin serum effects in islets of Langerhans' of chick embryo. Arch. Path. **77,** 107 (1964).

BLUMENTHAL, H. G., GOLDENBERG, S., BERNS, A. W.: The pathology and pathogenesis of the disseminated angiopathy of diabetes mellitus. Diabetes **14,** 309 (1965).

BORDUAS, A. G., GRABAR, P.: L'hémagglutination passive dans la recherche des anticorps antiprotéiques. Ann. Inst. Pasteur **84,** 903 (1953).

BOULIN, R., CHIMÈNES, H., TOURNEUR, R.: Etude de 14 cas de lipodystrophies insuliniques. Presse méd. **60,** 1024 (1952).

Boulin, R., Lapresle, Cl., Guéniot, M., Lapresle, J.: Périartérite noueuse apparue chez un diabétique quelques mois après une période d'insulino-résistance sévère. Presse méd. **63**, 1433 (1955).

Boyden, S. V.: Fixation of bacterial products by erythrocytes treated with tannic acid and subsequent haemagglutination by anti-protein sera. J. exp. Med. **93**, 107 (1951).

— Cytophilic antibody. In: Cell-bound Antibodies. Conf. Nat. Acad. Scien. Proc. ed. by B. Ammos and H. Koprowski. Wistar Inst. Press, Philadelphia 1963, p. 7.

— Cytophilic antibody in guinea pigs with delayed type hypersensitivity. Immunology **7**, 474 (1964).

— Sorkin, E.: The adsorption of antibody and antigen by spleen cells in vitro. Immunology **3**, 272 (1960).

— — The adsorption of antibody and antigen by spleen cells in vitro. Some further experiments. Immunology **4**, 244 (1961).

Brown, E. E.: Infectious origin of juvenile diabetes. Arch. Pediat. **73**, 191 (1956).

Brunfeldt, K. (1966) cited by Devlin (1968).

— Deckert, T.: Antibodies in the pig against pig insulin. Acta Endocr. **47**, 367 (1964).

Burnet, F. M.: The new approach to immunology. New Engl. J. Med. **264**, 24 (1961).

Carsten, M. E., Eisen, H. N.: The specific interaction of some dinitrobenzenes with rabbit antibody to dinitrophenyl-bovine gamma globulin. J. Amer. Soc. Chem. **77**, 1273 (1955).

Cawley, M. J., Browne, D. S.: Insulin resistance and thrombocytopenic purpura occurring in the same patient. Brit. J. Clin. Pract. **24**, 169 (1970).

Cerasi, E., Hogeman, O., Luft, R., Porath, J., Roovete, A.: Insulin antibodies: Description of specific serum protein localization in a patient with insulin resistant diabetes. Diabetologia **2**, 45 (1966).

Chadwick, C. S., McEntegart, M. G., Nairn, R. C.: Fluorescent protein tracing: a simple alternative to fluorescein. Lancet **1958 a I**, 412.

— — — Fluorescent protein tracers: a trial of new fluorochromes and the development of an alternative to fluorescein. Immunology **1**, 315 (1958 b).

Chance, R. E., Ellis, R. M., Bromer, W. W.: Porcine proinsulin: characterization and amino acid sequence. Science **161**, 165 (1968).

Chao, P. Y., Karam, J. H., Grodsky, G. M.: Insulin I-131 binding in serum from normal and diabetic subjects by ultrazentrifugation and gel-filtration. Diabetes **14**, 27 (1965).

Chase, M. W.: Cellular transfer of cutaneous hypersensitivity to tuberculin. Proc. Soc. Biol. Med. **59**, 134 (1945).

Clark, C., Munoz, J.: Delayed hypersensitivity to insulin and its component polypeptide chains. J. Immunol. **105**, 574 (1970).

Cole, L.: Diabetes mellitus in children. Lancet **1**, 947 (1934).

COLWELL, A. R., WEIGER, R. W.: Inhibition of Insulin Action by Serum Gamma Globulin. J. Lab. Clin. Med. **47,** 844 (1956).

CONSTAM, G. R.: Thrombocytopenic purpura as a probable manifestation of insulin allergy. Diabetes **5,** 121 (1956).

COOMBS, R. R. A., LACHMANN, P. J.: Immunological reactions at the cell surface. Brit. Med. Bull. **24,** 113 (1968).

— GELL, P. G. H.: Diagnostic and analytical in vitro methods. In: Clinical aspects of immunity. Eds.: P. G. H. GELL and R. R. A. COOMBS. Oxford and Edinburgh: Blackwell Scientific Publications 1968, p. 3.

COONS, A. H., KAPLAN, M. H.: Localization of antigen in tissue cells. II. Improvement on a method for the detection of antigen by means of a fluorescent antibody. J. Exp. Med. **91,** 1 (1950).

— LEDUC, E. H., KAPLAN, M. H.: Localization of antigen in tissue cells: VI. The fate of injected foreign proteins in the mouse. J. exp. Med. **93,** 173 (1951).

— — CONOLLY, J. M.: Studies on antibody production. I. A method for the histochemical demonstration of specific antibody and its application to a study of the hyperimmune rabbit. J. exp. Med. **102,** 49 (1955).

CREUTZFELDT, W., KERN, E., KÜMMERLE, F., SCHUMACHER, J.: Die radikale Entfernung der Bauchspeicheldrüse beim Menschen. Indikationen, Ergebnisse, Folgeerscheinungen. Erg. Inn. Med. Kinderheilk. **16,** 79 (1961).

CRUCHAUD, A.: Personal information by Prof. RENOLD (1966).

CUNNINGHAM, N. F., PATTERSON, D. S., WRIGHT, P. H.: Acute insulin deficiency provoked in sheep and cows by single injections of anti-insulin serum. J. Physiol. **169,** 137 (1963).

CUNNINGHAM, J. A.: A method of increased sensitivity for detecting single antibody forming cells. Nature **207,** 1107 (1965).

— SMITH, J. B., MERCER, E. H.: Antibody formation by single cells from lymph nodes and efferent lymph of sheep. J. exp. Med. **124,** 701 (1966).

DAHL, L. (1950) cited by HANSEN, Allergie 1957.

DAVID, J. R.: Macrophage inhibition. Fed. Proc. **27,** 6 (1968).

— AL ASKARI, S., LAWRENCE, H. S., THOMAS, L.: Delayed hypersensitivity in vitro. I. The specificity of inhibition of cell migration by antigens. J. Immunol. **93,** 264 (1964).

DAWEKE, H.: Klinik der Insulinresistenz. Dtsch. med. Wschr. **91,** 973 (1966).

DECKERT, T.: Insulin antibodies. Munksgaard. Copenhagen 1964.

— (1966 and 1968) personal communications.

— GRUNDAHL, E.: 5th annual meeting of Scand. Diabetes Assoc. Kopenhagen, 1969. Diabetologia **5,** 425 (1969) Abstr.

DEPISCH, F., HASENÖRL, R,: Experimentelle Untersuchungen über die Insulinresistenz beim Diabetes mellitus. Z. ges. exp. Med. **58,** 110 (1928).

DEVEY, M., CARTER, D., SANDERSON, C. J., COOMBS, R. R. A.: IgD antibody to insulin. The Lancet II, 1280 (1970).

DEVLIN, J. G.: Evidence for the existence of an IgM immunoglobulin to insulin. Irish J. med. Sci. 6th series. No. **491,** 507 (1966).

DEVLIN, J. G.: Hormone resistance and hypersensitivity. Clinical aspects of immunity. Eds.: P. G. H. GELL and R. R. A. COOMBS, Oxford and Edinburgh: Blackwell Scientific Publications 1968, p. 672.

— O'DONOVAN, D. K.: Association of acute local reactions to insulin with an insulin-binding gamma I M antibody. J. Clin. Path. **18,** 356 (1965).

— — Preferential Beef/Pork Insulin Binding Capacity. Radioimmunoelectrophoretic and Chromatographic Data in Patients with Dermal Reactions to Insulin. Diabetes **15,** 790 (1966).

DIENES and SCHÖNHEIT (1929) cited by DIENES (1930).

DIENES, L.: The first manifestation of the developing hypersensitivitiness. Proc. Soc. Exp. Biol. Med. **28,** 75 (1930).

DITSCHUNEIT, H., KAPP, H., FAULHABER, J. D., PFEIFFER, E. F., SCHÖFFLING, K.: Über Nachweis und klinische Bedeutung von Insulinantikörpern bei Insulinresistenten. 9. Symp. Dtsch. Ges. Endocr. Wiesbaden 1962. Berlin-Göttingen-Heidelberg: Springer 1963, p. 186.

— FEDERLIN, K.: Beitrag zur Pathogenese der Insulinresistenz. Dtsch. med. Wschr. **91,** 853 (1966).

— HINZ, M., FAULHABER, J. D.: Vergleichende quantitative Untersuchungen über Antikörper gegen Proinsulin und Insulin im Blut bei insulinbehandelten Diabetikern. 1. Tagg. Ges. f. Immunologie. Freiburg 1969. European J. Immunol. 1970, Abstr. p. 12.

DOLOVICH, J., SCHNATZ, J. D., REISMAN, R. E., YAGI, Y., ARBESMAN, C.: Insulin allergy and insulin resistance. J. Allergy **46,** 127 (1970).

DORÉ, C. F., BALFOUR, B. M.: Device for preparing cell spreads. Immunology **9,** 403 (1965).

DUFFUS, W. P. H., ALLEN, D.: A study of the ontogeny of specific immune responsiveness among circulating leucocytes in the chicken. Immunology **16,** 337 (1969).

EISEN, H. N., KARUSH, F.: Significance of valence in antibody interactions. J. Allergy **20,** 393 (1949).

ENGBRING, N. H., ARKINS, J. A., LENNON, E. J.: Insulin allergy and insulin resistance. J. Allergy **33,** 62 (1962).

ENGLESSON, G., NIELSSON, S. B.: Insulin antibodies in juvenile diabetes. Acta paediat. **51,** 433 (1962).

FARRELL, H. W., HAND, A. M., NEWCOMB, A. L.: Infantile diabetes. Diabetes **2,** 85 (1953).

FEDERLIN, K.: Autoimmunphänomene bei Erkrankungen endokriner Drüsen. Klin. Wschr. **47,** 337 (1969).

— Untersuchungen über die Antigenität von Insulin, Proinsulin und verwandten Proteinen am Meerschweinchen mit der passiven kutanen Anaphylaxie. Proinsulin und verwandte Proteine, Monokomponentinsulin. Arbeitsgespräch. Novo. Mainz 1970.

— HEINEMANN, G., GIGLI, I., DITSCHUNEIT, H.: Antigenbindung durch zirkulierende Leukocyten bei der verzögerten lokalen Insulinallergie. Dtsch. med. Wschr. **91,** 814 (1966).

FEDERLIN, K., KRIEGBAUM, D., FLAD, H. D.: Lymphocytentransformation in vitro bei verschiedenen Formen der Insulinallergie. Therapiewoche **45**, 2042 (1968).

— — — Experimentelle Untersuchungen zur verzögerten Insulinallergie. Verh. Dtsch. Ges. Inn. Med. **75**, 708 (1969).

— BIEDERMANN, M., PFEIFFER, E. F.: Antikörperbildende Zellen im Blut nach Sensibilisierung mit Insulin. Z. Immun.-Forsch. **138**, 141 (1969).

— DITSCHUNEIT, H., PFEIFFER, E. F.: Insulinallergie und Insulinresistenz. In: Handbuch des Diabetes mellitus. Hrsg.: E. F. PFEIFFER u. Mitarb. München: J. Lehmanns Verlag 1971 (in press).

— GIGLI, J.: Immunzytologische Aspekte der Antikörperbildung gegen Insulin. In: Allergie und Immunitätsforschung. II. Ed. by A. HEYMER and W. GRONEMEYER. Stuttgart: F. K. Schattauer 1968, p. 47.

— HEINEMANN, G.: Methods for the production of antibodies against low-molecular proteohormones. Symposion on Immunological methods in Endocrinology, Ulm 1970. Hormone and metabolic research (in press).

— RENOLD, A. E., PFEIFFER, E. F.: Antigen-binding leucocytes in patients and in insulin-sensitized animals with delayed insulin allergy. Immunopathology Vth Int. Symposium. Ed. by P. A. MIESCHER and P. GRABAR. Basel/Stuttgart: Schwabe & Co. Publ. 1968, p. 107.

— KRIEGBAUM, D., HEINEMANN, G., FLAD, H. D., PFEIFFER, E. F.: Experimental studies in animals on the antigenicity of insulin, of A and B chains and of fragments of synthetic insulin in terms of delayed immunoreactivity to insulin. Diabetologia **6**, 44 (1970) (Abstr.).

FITCH, F. W., WISSLER, R. W.: The Histology of Antibody Production. In: Immunological diseases. Ed. by M. SAMTER and H. L. ALEXANDER. London: Churchill 1965, p. 65.

FOTHERGILL, J. E.: Fluorochroms and their conjugation with proteins. In: Fluorescent protein tracing. Ed. by R. C. NAIRN. Edinburgh and London: E. & S. Livingstone Ltd. 1964 a.

— Properties of conjugated serum proteins. In: Fluorescent protein tracing. Ed. by R. C. NAIRN. Edinburgh and London: E. & S. Livingstone Ltd. 1964 b, p. 59.

FRASER, R., HARTOG, M.: Immunological studies with human growth hormone. In: Ciba Foundation Colloquia on Endocrinology **14**, 105 (1962).

FREEDMAN, S. O., TURCOTTE, R., FISH, A. J., SEHON, A. H.: The in vitro detection of cell-fixed hemagglutinating antibodies to tuberculin purified protein derivatives in humans. J. Immunol. **90**, 52 (1963).

FREI, P. C., CRUCHAUD, S., VANOTTI, A.: Allergie a l'insuline de type cellulaire. Rev. Franc. Études Clin. et Biol. **10**, 1083 (1965).

FREYTAG, G., MITSCHKE, H., KLÖPPEL, G.: Immunpathologische Untersuchungen zur experimentellen Insulitis. Verh. Dtsch. Ges. Path. **54**, 290 (1970).

— MENKE, B.: Latenter Diabetes mellitus bei Meerschweinchen während der aktiven Immunisierung gegen Fremdinsulin. 16. Symp. Dtsch. Ges. Endokrinologie. Berlin-Heidelberg-New York: Springer 1970, p. 65.

FROESCH, E. R., BÜRGI, H., RAMSEIER, E. B., BALLY, P., LABHART, A.: Antibody suppressible and non suppressible insulin like activities in human serum and their physiological significance. An insulin assay with adipose tissue of increased precision and specificity. J. Clin. Invest. **42,** 1816 (1963).

FUJI, G., NELSON, R. A.: Cross-reactivity and transfer of antibody in transplantation immunity. J. Exp. Med. **118,** 1037 (1963).

GARVIN, J. E.: Factors affecting the adhesiveness of human leucocytes and platelets in vitro. J. Exp. Med. **114,** 51 (1961).

GELL, P. G., BENACERRAF, B.: Delayed hypersensitivity to simple protein antigens. In: Advances in Immunology. Ed. by. W. H. TALIAFERRO and J. H. HUMPHREY. New York: Academic Press 1961, Vol. **1,** p. 319.

GEPTS, W.: Pathological anatomy of the pancreas in juvenile diabetes mellitus. Diabetes **14,** 619 (1965).

— Morphologie des Inselapparates beim Diabetes des Menschen. Verh. dtsch. Ges. inn. Med. 1966. München: J. F. Bergmann 1967, S. 834.

GILLISSEN, G.: Die fluoreszenzserologische Darstellung einer Komplementbindung durch zellständige Antikörper bei der Tuberkulose. Z. Hyg. Infekt.-Kr. **150,** 194 (1964).

— La définition sérologique des anticorps sessiles par rapport à la réaction tuberculinique. Rev. Immunol. (Paris) **27,** 43 (1963).

GLASSBERG, B. Y., SOMOGYI, M., TAUSSIG, A. E.: Diabetes mellitus. Report of a case refractory to insulin. Arch. Int. Med. **40,** 676 (1927).

GLIEMANN, J. (1967) cited by STEINER, HALLUND, RUBENSTEIN, CHO and BAYLISS (1968).

— MOODY, A. J. (1968) cited by STEINER, HALLUND, RUBENSTEIN, CHO and BAYLISS (1968).

GOETZ, F. C., GREENBERG, B. S., ELLIS, J., MEINERT, C.: A simple immunoassay for insulin: application to human and dog plasma. J. Clin. Endocr. Metabol. **23,** 1237 (1963).

GOLDNER, M. G., RICKETTS, H. T.: Insulin allergy: A report of eight cases with generalized symptoms. J. Clin. Endocrin. **2,** 595 (1942).

GREGOR, W. H., MARTIN, J. M., WILLIAMSON, J. R., LACY, P. E., KIPNIS, D. M.: A study of the diabetic syndrome produced in rats by anti-insulin serum. Diabetes **12,** 73 (1963).

GRIEBLE, H. C.: Renal lesions induced by heterologous insulin. An example of foreign protein nephritis. J. Lab. clin. Med. **56,** 8129 (1960).

GRODSKY, G. M.: Production of autoantibodies to insulin in man and rabbits. Diabetes **14,** 396 (1965).

— FORSHAM, P. H.: An immunochemical assay of total extractable insulin in man. J. Clin. Invest. **39,** 1070 (1960).

— FELDMAN, R., TORESON, W. E., LEE, J. C.: Diabetes mellitus in rabbits immunized with insulin. Diabetes **15,** 579 (1966).

GUNDERSEN, E.: Is diabetes of infectious origin? J. Infect. Dis. **41,** 197 (1927).

GUTHRIE, R. A., WOMACK, W.: Insulin resistance in diabetes in juveniles. Pediatrics **40**, 642 (1967).

HAGEN, H., HAGEN, W., HEINSEN, H. A., OLTERS, E. SCHEFFLER, H.: Experimentelle Untersuchungen über die Hautverträglichkeit von Insulinpräparaten. Dtsch. med. Wschr. **83**, 1480 (1958).

— — Experimentelle Untersuchungen über die Hautverträglichkeit von Insulinpräparaten. Ärztl. Forsch. **11**, 578 (1959).

HALES, C. N., RANDLE, P. J.: Immunoassay of insulin by isotopic dilution. Biochem. J. **84**, 79 (1962).

HALIKIS, D. N., ARQUILLA, E. R.: Studies on the Physical, Immunolocigal and Biological Properties of Insulin Conjugates with Fluorescein-Isothiocyanate. Diabetes **10**, 142 (1961).

HALPERN, B., KY, N., AMACHE, N.: Diagnosis of drug allergy in vitro with the lymphocyte transformation test. J. Allergy **40**, 168 (1967).

HANSEN, K.: Arzneimittel-Allergie. In: Allergie. Stuttgart: G. Thieme 1957, p. 395.

— EYER, H. D.: Klinische Studien über allergische Krankheiten und Insulinallergie. Dtsch. Arch. klin. Med. **174**, 133 (1933).

HARRIS, J. I., SANGER, F., NAUGHTON, M. A.: Species differences in insulin. Arch. Biochem. **65**, 427 (1956).

HAUROWITZ, F.: Chemistry and Biology of Protein. New York: Academic Press 1950, p. 284.

HEINEMANN, G.: Die Antigenbindung durch sensibilisierte Blutzellen bei der verzögerten Insulinallergie. Thesis Universität Ulm, 1971.

— FEDERLIN, K.: Antigenbindung durch sensibilisierte Zellen bei delayed hypersensitivity. 1. Sympos. über Leukocytenkulturen. Marburg 1969 (unpublished).

— KRIEGBAUM, D., FEDERLIN, K.: Untersuchungen über „zellständige" und humorale Antikörper bei der Insulinallergie. 1. Donausymposion über Diabetes mellitus. Wien 27./28. 6. 1969. Wien: Verlag der Wiener Medizinischen Akademie 1970, p. 397.

HEREMANS, J. F., VAERMAN, J. P.: β-2A-Globulin as a possible carrier of allergic reaginic activity. Nature **193**, 1091 (1962).

HINKE, H., STEINHILBER, S., SCHMIDT, D., KERP, L.: Quantitative Untersuchungen zur Antikörperbindung von Rinderinsulin und Rinderproinsulin in Seren insulinbehandelter Diabetiker. 76. Verh. Dtsch. Ges. Inn. Med. J. F. Bergmann, München 1970, p. 375.

HIRATA, Y., BLUMENTHAL, H. T.: Precipitation of insulin with sera of insulintreated guinea pigs and rabbits. J. Lab. Clin. Med. **60**, 194 (1962).

HJORT, T., BEUTNER, E. H., WITEBSKY, E.: Uptake of labelled antigens by lymphocytes of rabbits with delayed hypersensitivity reactions. Int. Arch. Allergy **33**, 337 (1968).

HOPKINS, F., WORMALL, A.: Phenyl isocyanate protein compounds and their immunological properties. Biochem. J. **27**, 740 (1933).

HORINO, M., YU, S. Y., BLUMENTHAL, H. T.: Studies on experimental insulin immunity. I. Dynamics of insulin immunity in the guinea pig. Diabetes **15,** 812 (1966).

HULLIGER, L., SORKIN, E.: Formation of specific antibody by circulating cells. Immunology **9,** 391 (1965).

HUMPHREY, J. H., WHITE, R. G.: Immunology for students of medicine. 2nd Edition. Oxford: Blackwell 1964, p. 300.

— — Immunology for students of medicine. Oxford and Edinburgh: Blackwell 1970, p. 135.

ISHIARA, Y., SAITO, T., ITO, Y., FUJINO, M.: Structure of sperm- and seiwhal insulins and their breakdown by whal pepsin. Nature **181,** 1468 (1958).

ISHIZAKA, K., ISHIZAKA, T., HORNBROOK, M. M.: Physicochemical properties of reaginic antibody. V. Correlation of reaginic activity with E globulin antibody. J. Immunol. **97,** 840 (1966).

ISHIZAKA, K., TOMIOKA, H., ISHIZAKA, T.: Mechanisms of passive sensitization. I. Presence of IgE and IgG molecules on human leucocytes. J. Immunol. **105,** 1459 (1970).

JERNE, N. K., NORDIN, A. A.: Plaque formation in agar by single antibody producing cells. Science **140,** 405 (1963).

— — HENRY, C.: The agar-plaque technique for recognizing antibody producing cells. Conference on cellbound antibody. Eds. AMOS and KOPROWSKI. Wistar Institute Press 1963, p. 109.

JOHN, H. J.: Diabetes mellitus in children; review of 500 cases. J. Pediat. **35,** 723 (1949).

JONES, T. D., MOTE, J. R.: Phases of foreign protein sensitization in human beings. N. Engl. J. Med. **210,** 120 (1934).

JONES, V. E., CUNLIFFE, A. C.: A precipitating antibody to insulin. Nature **192,** 136 (1961).

JORPES, J. I.: Recrystallized insulin for diabetic patients with insulin allergy. Arch. Int. Med. **83,** 363 (1949).

JOSLIN, E., GRAY, H., ROOT, R.: Insulin in Hospital and Home. J. metab. Res. **2,** 651 (1922).

KALLEE, E.: Über ^{131}J-signiertes Insulin. Z. Naturforsch. 7 B, 661 (1952).

KASEMIR, H., PAULUS, U., STEINHILBER, S., KERP, L.: Antikörperbindung von Rinder- und Schweineinsulin. 3. Tagung Dtsch. Diabetes-Ges. Göttingen 1968. Abst. diabetol. (Novo) p. 9, 1968.

KAY, K., RIEKE, W. O.: Tuberculin hypersensitivity: studies with radioactive antigen and mononuclear cells. Science **139,** 487 (1963).

KEARNEY, R., HALLIDAY, W. J.: Enumeration of antibody forming cells in the peripheral blood of immunized rabbits. J. Immunol. **95,** 109 (1964).

KEHRER, F. A.: Die Lipodystrophie. Stuttgart: G. Thieme 1949.

KERP, L.: Einfache Methoden zum Nachweis insulinneutralisierender Antikörper. Rundtischgespräch: Therapieprobleme bei Insulinresistenz. 74. Kongr. Dtsch. Ges. Inn. Med. 1968 (unpublished).

KERP, L., STEINHILBER, S., KIELING, F., CREUTZFELDT, W.: Klinische und experimentelle Untersuchungen zur Insulinallergie und Insulinresistenz. Dtsch. Med. Wsch. **90**, 806 (1965).

— — KASEMIR, H.: Ein Verfahren zum Nachweis insulinbindender Antikörper durch Differentialadsorption. Klin. Wschr. **44**, 560 (1966).

— KASEMIR, H., KIELING, F.: Insulinbindende Antikörper und Insulinbedarf bei Diabetikern. Klin. Wschr. **46**, 376 (1968).

— STEINHILBER, S., KASEMIR, H.: Besitzt die Proinsulinverunreinigung kommerzieller Insulinpräparate Bedeutung für die Stimulierung von Insulinantikörpern? Klin. Wschr. **48**, 884 (1970).

— — SCHMIDT, D. D.: Vergleichende Analyse der gegen Rinderproinsulin und Rinderinsulin gebildeten Antikörper. FEBS-Letters **8**, 157 (1970).

KIMMELSTIEL, B., WILSON, C.: cited by ANDERSON (1953). Am. J. Path. **12**, 45 (1936).

KITAGAWA, M., ONOUE, K., OKAMURA, Y., ANAI, M., YAMAMURA, Y.: cited by POPE (1966). J. Biochem. (Tokyo) **48**, 43 (1960 a).

— — — — — cited by POPE (1966). J. Biochem. (Tokyo) **48**, 483 (1960 b).

KOPROWSKI, H., FERNANDES, M. V.: Autosensitization in vitro. J. exp. Med. **116**, 467 (1962).

KREMER, H. U.: Juvenile diabetes as a sequel of mumps. Amer. J. Med. **3**, 257 (1947).

KRIEGBAUM, D., FEDERLIN, K.: Experimental investigations of the delayed immune response to insulin fractions. Diabetologia **6**, 78 (1970) (Abstr.).

KULPE, W.: Hautnekrosen bei der Insulinbehandlung durch Surfen-Überempfindlichkeit. Münch. med. Wschr. **100**, 998 (1958).

LACHNIT, V., WIEDERMANN, G.: Immunologische Untersuchungen bei Insulinallergie. Z. Immun.-Forsch. **122**, 216 (1961).

LACY, P. E.: Electron microscopy of the normal islets of Langerhans; studies in the dog, rabbit, guinea pig and rat. Diabetes **6**, 498 (1957).

— Electron microscopic and fluorescent antibody studies on islets of Langerhans. Exp. Cell. Res. Suppl. **7**, 296 (1959).

— DAVIES, J.: Preliminary studies on the demonstration of insulin in the islets by fluorescent antibody technic. Diabetes **6**, 354 (1957).

— — Demonstration of insulin in mammalian pancreas by the fluorescent antibody method. Stain technol. **34**. 85 (1959).

— WRIGHT, D. H.: Allergic interstitial pancreatitis in rats injected with guinea pig anti-insulin serum. Diabetes **14**, 634 (1965).

LANDSTEINER, K., CHASE, M. W.: Experiments on transfer of cutaneous sensitivity to simple chemical compounds. Proc. Soc. exp. Biol. (N. Y.) **49**, 688 (1942).

LAPRESLE, C., GRABAR, P.: Mise en évidence d'une impureté antigenique dans les preparations d'insuline et d'anticorps correspondants dans le sérum de diabetiques traités par l'insuline. Rev. Franc. Étud. Clin. Biol. **2**, 1025 (1957).

LAWRENCE, H. S.: The cellular transfer of cutaneous hypersensitivity to tuberculin in man. Proc. Soc. exp. Biol. (N. Y.) **71**, 516 (1949).

— The transfer in humans of delayed skin sensitivity to streptococcal M-substance and to tuberculin. J. clin. Invest. **34**, 219 (1955).

— Some biological and immunological properties of transfer factor. In: Cellular aspects of immunity. A Ciba Foundation Symposium. London: J. & A. Churchill 1960, p. 243.

LAYTON, L. L., LEE, S., YAMANAKA, E.: Allergen testing on monkeys passively sensitized by Hay Fever and Asthma Reagins of Human Sera. Nature **193**, 988 (1962).

— PANZANI, R., GREENE, F. C., CORSE, J. W.: Atopic hypersensitivity to a protein of the Green Coffee Bean and absence of allergic reactions to Chlorogenic Acid, Low-Molecular-Weight components of green coffee, or to roasted coffee. Int. Arch. Allergy **28**, 1 (1965).

LECOMPTE, P. M.: "Insulitis" in early juvenile diabetes. Arch. Path. **66**, 450 (1958).

— STEINKE, J., SOELDNER, J. S., RENOLD, A. E.: Changes in the islets of Langerhans in cows injected with heterologous and homologous insulin. Diabetes **15**, 586 (1966).

LEDUC, E. H., COONS, A. H., CONOLLY, J. M.: Studies on antibody production. II. The primary and secondary response in the popliteal lymph node of the rabbit. J. exp. Med. **102**, 61 (1955).

LERMAN, J.: Insulin resistance. The role of immunity in its production. Amer. J. Med. Soc. **207**, 354 (1944).

LEWIS, J. H.: The antigenic properties of insulin. J. Amer. J. Ass. **108**, 1336 (1937).

LINDERSTRÖM-LANG, K.: Symposion on peptide chemistry. Deuterium exchange between peptide and water. Chem. Soc. Spec. Publ. **2**, 1 (1955).

LINDLAY, H., ROLLETT, J. S.: An investigation of insulin structure by model building techniques. Biochem. Biophys. Acta **18**, 183 (1955).

LOVELESS, M. H., CANN, J. R.: Distribution of allergic and blocking activity in human serum protein fractionated by electrophoretic convection. Science **17**, 105 (1953).

— — Distribution of "blocking" antibody in human serum proteins fractionated by electrophoresis-convection. J. Immunol. **74**, 329 (1955).

LOW, B. V., EDSALL, J. T. E.: Aspects of protein structure. Currents in Biochem. Research, D. E. GREEN, Ed. Interscience, New York 1956, p. 378.

LOWELL, F. C.: Evidence for the existence of two antibodies for crystalline insulin. Proc. Soc. Exp. Biol. (N. Y.) **50**, 167 (1942).

— Immunologic studies in insulin resistance. I. Report of a case exhibiting variations in resistance and allergy to insulin. J. Clin. Invest. **23**, 225 (1944 a).

— Immunologic studies in insulin resistance. II. The presence of a neutralizing factor in the blood exhibiting some characteristics of an antibody. J. Clin. Invest. **23**, 233 (1944 b).

LOWELL, F. C.: Immunologic studies in insulin resistance. III. Measurement of an insulin antagonist in the serum of an insulin-resistant patient by the blood sugar curve method in mice. J. Clin. Invest. **26,** 57 (1947).

MAGER, A.: Personal Communication (1966).

MANCINI, A. M., ZAMPA, G. A., GEMINIANI, G. D., VECCHI, A.: Experimental nodular "diabetic-like" glomerulosclerosis in guinea pigs following long-acting, heterologous insulin immunization. Diabetologia 5, 155 (1969).

— — VECCHI, A., COSTANZI, G.: Histoimmunological techniques for detecting antiinsulin antibodies in human sera. Lancet **1965 I,** 1189.

MANN, C. B., SMITH, G. H.: The state of plasma insulin in guinea pigs with circulating antibodies to ox insulin. Biochem. J. **88,** 13 P (1963).

MARBLE, A.: Allergy and diabetes. In: JOSLIN, E. P., ROOT, H. F., WHITE, P., MARBLE, A.: The treatment of diabetes mellitus, 10. Edition. Philadelphia: Lea & Febiger 1959 a, p. 395.

— Disorders of the skin in diabetes. In: JOSLIN, E. P., ROOT, H. F., WHITE, P., MARBLE, A.: The treatment of diabetes mellitus, 10. Edition. Philadelphia: Lea & Febiger 1959 b, p. 592.

MARSH, J. B., HAUGAARD, N.: The effect of serum from insulin-resistant cases on the combination of insulin with the rat diaphragm. J. Clin. Invest. **31,** 107 (1952).

MARSHALL, J. D., EVELAND, W. C., SMITH, C. W.: Superiority of fluorescein-isothiocyanate (Riggs) for fluorescent-antibody technic with a modification of its application. Proc. Soc. exp. Biol. (N. Y.) **98,** 898 (1958).

MARTIN, W. P., MARTIN, H. E., LYSTER, R. W., STROUSE, S.: Insulin resistance. Critical survey of the literature with the report of a case. J. clin. Endocr. **1,** 387 (1941).

MAYERSBACH, H. VON: Immunhistologische Methoden in der Histochemie. In: Handbuch der Histochemie I/1. Allg. Methodik. Stuttgart: G. Fischer 1958.

— Immunhistologische Methoden in der Histochemie. In: Handbuch der Histochemie, I/2 (Ergänzungsbeitrag zu I/1). Stuttgart: G. Fischer 1966, S. 188.

— SCHUBERT, G.: Die unspezifischen Reaktionen zwischen markierten Seren und Geweben bei der immunhistologischen Technik. Acta histochem. **10,** 44 (1960).

— GROSSI, C. E. (1963): unpublished (cited by v. MAYERSBACH 1966).

MCDEVITT, H. O.: Delayed hypersensitivity to insulin in guinea pigs. Fed. Proc. **23,** 259 (1964).

— PETERS, J. H., POLARD, L. W., HARTER, J. G., COONS, A. H.: Purification and analysis of fluorescein-labeled antisera by column chromatography. J. Immunol. **90,** 634 (1963).

MCKAY, D. G., BENITSCHKE, K., CURTIS, G. W.: Infants of diabetic mothers. Histologic and histochemical observations on the pancreas. Obstet. Gynec. **2,** 133 (1953).

McMaster, P. D. (1953) cited by Uhr u. Finkelstein (1966).

Meade, R. C., Klitgaard, H. H.: A simplified method for immunoassay of human serum-insulin. J. nucl. Med. **3**, 407 (1962).

Melani, F., Ditschuneit, H., Bartelt, K. M., Friedrich, H., Pfeiffer, E. F.: Über die radioimmunologische Bestimmung von Insulin im Blut. Klin. Wschr. **43**, 1000 (1965).

— Rubenstein, A. H., Steiner, D. F.: Human serum proinsulin. J. clin. Invest. **49**, 497 (1970).

— — Oyer, P. E., Steiner, D. F.: Identification of Proinsulin and C-Peptide in Human Serum by a Specific Immunoassay. Proc. nat. Acad. Sci. (Wash.) **67**, 148 (1970).

Melin, K., Ursing, B.: Diabetes mellitus som Komplikatin till parotitis epidemica. Nord. Med. **60**, 1715 (1958).

Meyenburg, H. von: Über „Insulitis“ bei Diabetes. Schweiz. med. Wschr. **70**, 554 (1940).

Michel, H.: Insulin als Antigen. Eine klinisch-experimentelle Studie. Acta allerg. **16**, 1 (1961).

Miescher, Dixon, Waksman: cited by LeCompte et al. 1966.

Miller, J. M., Favour, C. B.: The lymphocytic origin of plasma factors responsible for hypersensitivity in vitro of the tuberculin type. J. exp. Med. **93**, 1 (1951).

Miller, R.: Tödliche anaphylaktische Reaktion nach Insulininjektion. Med. Welt **1962**, 2735.

Mitchison, N. A.: Immunological tolerance (ed. by M. Landy and W. Braun). New York 1969, p. 115.

Mohos, S. C., Henningar, G. R., Fogelman, J. A.: Insulin induced glomerulosclerosis in the rabbit. J. exp. Med. **118**, 667 (1963).

Moinat, P. S.: A quantitative estimation of antibodies to exogenous insulin in diabetic subjects. Diabetes **7**, 462 (1958).

Moloney, P. J., Coval, M.: Antigenicity of Insulin: diabetes induced by specific antibodies. Biochem. J. **59**, 179 (1955).

— Goldsmith, L.: On the antigenicity of insulin. Canad. J. Biochem. **35**, 79 (1957).

— Aprile, M. A.: On the antigenicity of insulin: Flocculation of insulin-antiinsulin. Canad. J. Biochem. Physiol. **37**, 793 (1959).

Morgan, C. R., Lazarow, A.: Immunoassay of insulin using a two-antibody system. Proc. Soc. exp. Biol. (N. Y.) **110**, 29 (1962).

Morse, J. H.: Rapid production and detection of insulin-binding antibodies in rabbits and guinea-pigs. Proc. Soc. exper. Biol. (N. Y.) **101**, 722 (1959).

— Correlation of insulin requirement with the concentration of insulin-binding antibody in two cases of insulin resistance. J. clin. Endocr. Metabol. **21**, 533 (1961).

— Heremans, J. F.: Correlation of insulin requirements with concentration of insulin-binding antibody and its papain-produced fragments. J. Lab. clin. Med. **59**, 892 (1962).

MOVAT, H. Z.: Antigen-Antikörper-Komplexe und allergische Entzündung. Verh. dtsch. path. Ges. **46,** 240 (1962).

NAIRN, R. C.: Immunological tracing: general considerations. In: Fluorescent protein tracing. Ed. by R. C. NAIRN. Edinburgh and London: E. & S. Livingstone Ltd. 1964, p. 103.

NELSON, R. A. jr.: The immune-adherence phenomenon: An immunologically specific reaction between microorganism and erythrocytes leading to enhanced phagocytosis. Science **118,** 735 (1953).

NICOL, D. S. H. W., SMITH, L. F.: Amino-acid sequence of human insulin. Nature (Lond.) **187,** 483 (1960).

NISONOFF, A., PRESSMAN, D.: Loss of precipitating activity of antibody without destruction of binding sites. J. Immunol. **81,** 126 (1958).

NOTA, N. A., LIACOPOULOS-BRIOT, M., STIFFEL, C., BIOZZI, G.: Immuno-cyto-adhérence: une methode simple et quantitative pour l'étude in vitro des cellules productrices d'anticorps. C. R. Acad. Sci. (Paris) **259,** 1277 (1964).

NOWELL, P. C.: Phytohaemagglutinin: An initiator of mitosis in cultures of normal human leucocytes. Cancer Res. **20,** 462 (1960).

OAKLEY, G. W., FIELD, J. B., SOWTON, G. E., RIGBY, B,. CUNLIFFE, A. C.: Action of prednisone in insulin-resistant diabetes. Brit. Med. J. **1,** 1601 (1959).

OBERDISSE, K.: Insulinresistenz und Diabetes mellitus. Dtsch. Arch. klin. Med. **193,** 247 (1948).

OGILVIE, R. F.: The endocrine pancreas in human and experimental diabetes. In: The Aetiology of Diabetes mellitus and its Complications. Ciba Foundation Colloquia on Endocrinology, Vol. 15. Ed. by M. P. CAMERON and M. O'CONNOR. London: Churchill 1964, p. 49.

ONCLEY, J. L., ELLENBOGEN, E., GITLIN, D., GURD, F. R. N.: Protein-protein interactions. J. Phys. Chem. **56,** 85 (1952).

OPIE, E. L.: On the relation of chronic interstitial pancreatitis to the islands of Langerhans and to diabetes mellitus. J. exp. Med. **5,** 397 (1900—1901).

ORTEGA, L. G., MELLORS, R. C.: Cellular sites of formation of gamma globulin. J. exp. Med. **106,** 627 (1957).

OVARY, Z.: Immediate reactions in the skin of experimental animals provoced by antibody antigen interaction. Progr. Allergy **5,** 459 (1958).

— Passive cutaneous anaphylaxis in the guinea pig: degree of reaction as a function of the quantitiy of antigen and antibody. Int. Arch. Allergy **14,** 18 (1959).

— Passive cutaneous anaphylaxis. In: Immunological Methods. Ed. by ACKROYD. Oxford: J. F. Blackwell 1964, p. 259.

OYER, P. E., CHO, S., STEINER, D. F.: Isolation and structure of human proinsulin C-peptide. Fed. Proc. **25,** 533 (1970).

PALEY, R. G., TUNBRIDGE, R. E.: Dermal reactions to insulin therapy. Diabetes **1,** 22 (1952).

PARKER, J. W., ELEVITCH, F. R., GRODSKY, G. M.: Binding of fluorescent insulin to intracellular antibodies in guinea-pigs immunized with insulin. Proc. Soc. exp. Biol. (N. Y.) **113,** 48 (1963).

PATTERSON, R., COLWELL, J. A., GREGOR, W. H., CARY, E.: Avian anti-insulin serum: a comparison of its immunologic and biologic activity with that of guinea pig and rabbit antisera. J. Lab. Clin. Med. **64,** 399 (1964).

— ROBERTS, M., PRUZANSKY, J. J.: Comparison of reaginic antibodies from three species. J. Immunol. **102,** 466 (1969).

PÁV, J., JEZKOVA, Z., SKRHA, F.: Insulin antibodies. Lancet **1963 II,** 221.

PEARMAIN, G., LYSETTE, R. R., FITZGERALD, P. H.: Tuberculin induced mitosis in peripheral blood leucocytes. Lancet **1963 I,** 637.

PEARSE, A. G. E.: Histochemistry-Theoretical and Applied. 2nd Ed. London: Churchill 1960, p. 137, 722.

PELTIER, A. P., KOURILSKY, R.: Etùde de la fixation d'antigenes proteiques par les cellules gangionaires de cobayes en etat hypersensibilité retardee pure. Ann. Inst. Pasteur. **110,** 813 (1966).

PENCHEV, I., ANDREW, D., DITZOV, S.: Insulin precipitating antibodies in insulin-treated and untreated diabetic patients. Diabetologia **4,** 164 (1968).

PFEIFFER, E. F.: Die Insulinresistenz. (Aktuelle Diagnostik.) Dtsch. med. Wschr. **91,** 314 (1966).

— Die Immunologie des Insulins. Verh. Dtsch. Ges. Inn. Med. 1966. München: J. F. Bergmann 1967, p. 811.

— DITSCHUNEIT, H.: Aktuelle Probleme der Diabetestherapie. Dtsch. med. Wschr. **87,** 2290 (1962).

— — FEDERLIN, K.: Die Immunologie des Insulins. In: Handbuch des Diabetes mellitus. Ed. by E. F. PFEIFFER. München: J. F. Lehmanns Verlag 1969, p. 155.

PLOTZ, P., TALLAL, N.: Fractionation of splenic antibody forming cells on glass bead columns. J. Immunol. **99,** 1236 (1967).

POETSCHKE, G., UEHLEKE, H., KILLISCH, L.: Untersuchungen mit fluorescein-markierten Antikörpern. I. Allgemeines und Methodisches. Z. Immun.-Forsch. **114,** 393 (1957).

POPE, C. G.: The Immunology of Insulin. Advances Immunol. **5,** 209 (1966).

PORTER, R. D., HARTMAN, C. R.: Arthus reactions from insulin. Association with lupus erythematosus cell phenomena. J. Amer. Med. Ass. **214,** 1884 (1970).

PRAUSNITZ, C., KÜSTNER, H.: Studien über die Überempfindlichkeit. Zbl. Bakt. **86,** 160 (1921).

PRESSMAN, D., CAMPBELL, D. H., PAULING, L.: Complement fixation with simple substances containing two or more haptenic groups. Proc. nat. Acad. Sci. **28,** 77 (1942).

RABINOWITZ, Y.: Separation of lymphocytes, polymorphonuclear leucocytes on glass bead columns including tissue observations. Blood **23,** 811 (1964).

RAFFEL, S.: Delayed hypersensitivity (cellular). In: Immunological diseases. Ed. by M. SAMTER and H. L. ALEXANDER. London: Churchill 1965, p. 146.

— NEWEL, J. M.: Delayed hypersensitivity induced by antigen-antibody complexes. J. exp. Med. **108,** 823 (1958).

RAMSEIER, E. B., FROESCH, E. R., BALLY, P., LABHART, A.: Seruminsulinbestimmung am Fettgewebe in vitro: Beeinflussung durch andere Hormone. „Freie" und „gebundene" Insulinaktivität. 4. Kongr. Intern. Diab. Foed. Genf 1961. Ed. Méd. Hyg. Vol. I, p. 643.

RAUSCH-STROOMANN, I. G., SAUER, H.: Zur Frage der Insulinresistenz durch Antikörperbildung. Klin. Wschr. **31,** 551 (1953).

RENOLD, A. E., SOELDNER, J. S., STEINKE, J.: Immunological studies with homologous and heterologous pancreatic insulin in the cow. Ciba Foundation Colloq. Endocr. London: Churchill 1964, Vol. 15, p. 122.

— STEINKE, J., SOELDNER, J. S., GONET, A., LECOMPTE, P.: Insulite experimentale chez la genisse. Fourth Internat. Symposium on Immunopathology. Eds.: MIESCHER and GRABAR. Basel: Benno Schwabe 1965, p. 349.

— GONET, A. E., VECCHIO, D.: Immunopathology of the endocrine pancreas. In: Textbook of Immunopathology. Eds.: P. A. MIESCHER and H. J. MÜLLER-EBERHARD, Vol. II. p. 959. New York and London: Grune and Stratton 1969, p. 595.

RICH, A. R., LEWIS, M. R.: Mechanisms of allergy in tuberculosis. Proc. Soc. exp. Biol. (N. Y.) **25,** 596 (1928).

RICHARDSON, R.: Complement fixation with insulin as antigen. Proc. Soc. exper. Biol. (N. Y.) **38,** 874 (1938).

RINDERKNECHT, H.: A new technique for the fluorescent labelling of proteins. Experientia (Basel) **16,** 430 (1960).

— Ultra-rapid fluorescent labelling of proteins. Nature (Lond.) **193,** 167 (1962).

RITTS, R. E., FAVOUR, C. B.: In vivo uptake of isotope tagged tuberculin by leucocytes. J. Immunol. **75,** 209 (1955).

RIVERA, J. U., TORO-GOYCO, E., MATOS, M. C.: Molecular sieve in the study of plasma proteins. Amer. J. med. Sci. **249,** 371 (1965).

ROBINSON, B. H. B., WRIGHT, P. H.: Guinea-pig anti-insulin serum. J. Clin. Physiol. **155,** 302 (1961).

ROITT, I. M., GREAVES, M. F., TORRIGIANI, G., BROSTOFF, J., PLAYFAIR, J. H. L.: The cellular basis of immunological responses. Lancet **1969 II,** 367.

ROMEIS, B.: Mikroskopische Technik. München: R. Oldenbourg 1948.

ROSE, C., BARRON, J.: Anaphylactic shock as a complication of insulin coma therapy. Brit. med. J. **1955 I,** 583.

ROSE, N., BROWN, R. C.: Cytophilic antibody. Fed. Proc. **21,** 44 (1962).

ROSENAU, W., MOON, H. D.: Lysis of homologous cells by sensitized lymphocytes in tissue culture. J. nat. Cancer Inst. **27,** 471 (1961).

ROSSELIN, G., TCHOBROUTSKY, G., ASSAN, R., LELLOUCH, L., DOLAIS, J., DEROT, M.: Étude quantitative d'anticorps humains anti-insulines animales par la méthode Radio-Immunologique de BERSON et YALOW. Diabetologia **1,** 33 (1965).

RUBENSTEIN, A. H., CHO, S., STEINER, D. F.: Evidence for proinsulin in human urine and serum. Lancet **I,** 353 (1968).

RUBENSTEIN, A., STEINER, D. F., CHO, S., LAWRENCE, A. M., KISTEINS, L.: Immunological properties of bovine proinsulin and related fractions. Diabetes **18,** 598 (1969).

RUDY, A.: Urticaria and insulin resistance with reference to the relation of the skin to carbohydrate metabolism. New. Engl. J. Med. **204,** 791 (1931).

SAMOLS, E., JONES, V.: Insulin resistance and the relationship of human antibodies to insulin when measured by three different methods. First Annual Meeting of the European Association for the Study of Diabetes. Diabetologia **1,** 75 (1965) (Abstr.).

SANGER, F.: Chemistry of insulin; determination of the structure of insulin opens the way to greater understanding of life processes. Science **129,** 1340 (1959).

— Chemistry of insulin. Brit. Med. Bull. **16,** 183 (1960).

SELA, M.: Immunological studies with synthetic polypeptides. In: Advances in Immunology **5,** 29 (1966). Ed. by F. J. DIXON and J. HUMPHREY. Academic Press, London-New York.

— ARNON, R.: Studies on the chemical basis of the antigenicity of proteins. 1. Antigenicity of polypeptidyl gelatins. Biochem. J. **75,** 91 (1960 a).

— — Studies on the chemical basis of the antigenicity of proteins. 3. The role of rigidity in the antigenicity of polypeptidyl gelatines. Biochem. J. **77,** 394 (1960 b).

SENIOW, S.: Personal communication (1966).

SHAW, W. N., CHANCE, R. E.: Effect of porcine proinsulin in vitro on adipose tissue and diaphragm of the normal rat. Diabetes **17,** 737 (1968).

SHERMAN, W. B.: A case of coexisting insulin allergy and insulin resistance. J. Allergy **21,** 49 (1950).

SHIPP, J. C., CUNNINGHAM, R. W., RUSSEL, R. O., MARBLE, A.: Insulin resistance: clinical features, natural course and effects of adrenal steroid treatment. Medicine **44,** 165 (1965).

SILVERMAN, J. L.: Eosinophil infiltration in the pancreas of infants of diabetic mothers. A clinicopathological study. Diabetes **12,** 528 (1963).

SKOM, J. H., TALMAGE, D. W.: Non-precipitating insulin-antibodies. J. Clin. Invest. **37,** 783 (1958 a).

— — The role of non-precipitating insulin-antibodies in diabetes. J. Clin. Invest. **37,** 787 (1958 b).

SKOOG, W. A., BECK, W. S.: Studies on the fibrinogen, Dextran and Phytohaemagglutinin. Methods of isolating leucocytes. Blood **11,** 436 (1956).

SLATER, J. D. H., SAMAAN, N. A., FRASER, R., STILLMAN, D.: Immunologic studies with circulating insulin. Brit. med. J. **1961 I,** 1712.

SORKIN, E.: Cytophilic antibody. In: The immunologically competent cell. Ciba Foundation Study Group No. 16. Ed. by G. E. W. WOLSTENHOLME and J. KNIGHT. London: Churchill 1963, p. 38.

— RHODES, J. M., BOYDEN, S. V.: Antibody synthesis in relation to levels of humoral and cell fixed antibodies in rabbits. J. Immunol. **86,** 101 (1961).

— LANDY, M.: Antibody production by blood leucocytes. Experientia **21,** 677 (1965).

SPOONT, S., DYER, W. W.: Insulin-resistance associated with local and general allergy to insulin. J. Amer. med. Ass. **145,** 558 (1951).

SCHEFFLER, H.: Lokalisierte allergische Hautreaktionen mit Pigmentablagerung nach Insulininjektion. Medizinische 1955, p. 1409.

SCHEIFFARTH, F., FRENGER, W., MÖCKEL, G.: Serologische Studien über das Wesen der Insulin-Antikörper. Dtsch. med. Wschr. **84,** 177 (1959).

SCHIRREN, G. C.: Ein ungewöhnlicher Fall von lokaler Insulinanaphylaxie. Hautarzt **4,** 531 (1953).

SCHLICHTKRULL, J.: Insulin crystals. Copenhagen: Munksgaard 1953.

— Insuline: Allergien, Antikörper, Artspezifität und Antigencharakter. Medical Tribune **42,** 4 (1967).

— BRANGE, J., EGE, H., HALLUND, O., HEDING, L. G., JØRGENSEN, K., MARKUSSEN, J., STAHNKE, P., SUNDBY, F., VØLUND, AA.: Proinsulin und verwandte Proteine. Abstr. diabetol. (NOVO Service) 1969, p. 135.

— Proinsulin und verwandte Proteine — chemische und biologische Untersuchungen. 76. Tagg. Dtsch. Ges. Inn. Med. Wiesbaden 1970. J. F. Bergmann, München 1970, p. 14.

SCHMIDT, D. D., ARENS, A.: Proinsulin vom Rind. Isolierung, Eigenschaften und seine Aktivierung durch Trypsin. Hoppe Seyler's Z. phys. Chem. **349,** 1157 (1968).

SCHÖFFLING, K.: Insulinstoffwechsel des pankreaslosen Hundes. 12. Symp. Dtsch. Ges. Endokr., Wiesbaden 1966, p. 200. Berlin-Heidelberg-New York: Springer 1967.

SCHULTZ and DALE cited by HUMPHREY and WHITE.

SCHWARTSMAN, J., CRUSIUS, M. E., BEIRNE, D. P.: Diabetes mellitus in infants under one year of age. Amer. J. Dis. Child **74,** 587 (1947).

SCHWARTZ, P., KURUCZ, J., KURUCZ, A.: Fluorescence microscopy demonstration of cerebrovascular amyloid in presenile and senile states. J. Amer. Geriat. Soc. **13,** 199 (1965).

STAVITSKY, A. B., ARQUILLA, E. R.: Estimation of insulin and antibodies to insulin in vitro by haemagglutination and haemolysis of insulin-treated red cells and inhibition of these reactions. Fed. Proc. **12,** 461 (1953).

STEFFEN, C., ROSACK, M.: In vitro-demonstration of antiovalbumin specificity of lymph node cells in delayed type hypersensitivity. J. Immunol. **90,** 337 (1963).

STEIGERWALD, D., SPIELMANN, W.: Nachweis von Insulinantikörpern bei Diabetikern mit Insulinresistenz in Hämagglutinationstest und Coombstest. Klin. Wschr. **34,** 80 (1956).

STEIGERWALD, H., SPIELMANN, W., FRIES, H., GREBE, S. F.: Neue Untersuchungen über die Antigenwirkung des Insulins. Klin. Wschr. **38,** 973 (1960).

STEINER, L. A., EISEN, H. N.: The Nature of Antigen-Antibody-Interactions. In: Immunological diseases. Ed. by M. SAMTER and H. L. ALEXANDER. London: Churchill 1965, S. 122.

STEINER, D. F.: Evidence for a precursor in the biosynthesis of insulin. Trans. N. Y. Acad. Sci. Series II **30,** 60 (1967).

— OYER, P.: The biosynthesis of insulin and a probable precursor of insulin by a human islet cell adenoma. Proc. nat. Acad. Sci. U. S. **57,** 473 (1967).

— CUNNINGHAM, D., SPIGELMAN, L., ATEN, B.: Insulin biosynthesis: Evidence for a precursor. Science **157,** 697 (1967).

— CLARK, J. L.: The spontaneous reoxidation of reduced beef and rat proinsulins. Proc. nat. Acad. Sci. U. S. **60,** 622 (1968).

— HALLUND, O., RUBENSTEIN, A., CHO, S., BAYLISS, C.: Isolation and properties of proinsulin, intermediate forms and other minor components from crystalline bovine insulin. Diabetes **17,** 725 (1968).

— CLARK, J. L., NOLAN, C., RUBENSTEIN, A. H., MARGOLIASH, E., MELANI, F., OYER, P. E.: The biosynthesis of insulin and some speculations regarding the pathogenesis of human diabetes. Nobel Symposium 13. Ed. by E. CERASI and R. LUFT. Stockholm: Almquist & Wiksell 1970, p. 57.

STICKL, H., ENGELHARDT, J.: Die Leukocytolyse als Zeichen der spezifischen Reaktionsfähigkeit der Gewebe auf Vakzinevirus nach der Pockenschutzimpfung. Klinische, experimentelle und elektronenoptische Untersuchungen. Z. Hyg. Infekt. Kr. **151,** 111 (1965).

STOLL, R. W., TOUBER, J. L., ENSINCK, J. W., WILLIAMS, R. H.: Substances immunologically related to proinsulin or connecting peptide in swine plasma. Horm. Metab. Res. **2,** 153 (1970).

TIETZE, F., MORTIMORE, G. E., LOMAX, N. R.: Preparation and properties of fluorescent insulin derivatives. Biochem. Biophys. Acta **59,** 336 (1962).

TORESON, W. E., FELDMAN, R., LEE, J. C., GRODSKY, G. M.: Pathology of diabetes mellitus produced in rabbits by means of immunization with beef insulin. Amer. J. clin. Path. **42,** 531 (1964).

TORO-GOYCO, E., MARTINEZ-MALDONALD, M., MATOS, M.: Insulin antibodies: partial characterization by gel-filtration. Proc. Soc. exp. Biol. (N. Y.) **122,** 301 (1966).

TOUSSAINT, D., GEPTS, W.: Étude des lesions retiniennes, renales et insulinaires chez des chiens et des chats spontanement diebétiques. Abstr. 2. Tagung Europ. Ges. f. Diabetologie. Aarhus 1966, p. 118.

TUCKER, W. R., KLINK, D., GOETZ, F., ZALME, E., KNOWLES JR. H. C.: Insulin resistance and acanthosis nigricans. Diabetes **13,** 395 (1964).

TUFT, L.: Insulin hypersensitivitiness. — Immunologic considerations and case reports. Amer. J. med. Sci. **176,** 707 (1928).

TURK, J. L.: Some quantitative aspects of the uptake of antigens in vitro by the lymphocytes of hypersensitive guinea pigs. Int. Arch. Allergy **17**, 338 (1960).

— Delayed Hypersensitivity. Frontiers of Biology, Vol. 4. Amsterdam: North Holland Publ. Co. 1967.

VAZQUEZ, J. J.: Antibody and gamma globulin-forming cells as observed by the fluorescent antibody technique. Lab. Invest. **10**, 1120 (1961).

— Kinetics of Proliferation of Antibody Forming Cells. In: The Thymus in Immunobiology. Ed. by R. A. GOOD and A. E. GABRIELSEN. New York: P. B. Hoeber 1964, p. 298.

WAKSMAN, B. H.: A comparative histopathological study of delayed hypersensitivity reactions. In: Cellular aspects of immunity. Ciba Found Symposium. London: Churchill 1960, p. 280.

— Autoimmunization and the lesions of autoimmunity. Medicine **41**, 93 (1962).

WALKER, S. E.: cit. by MICHEL (1961). U.S. Vet. Bur. Med. Bull. **2**, 2700 (1926).

WARREN, S., ROOT, H. F.: The pathology of diabetes with special reference to pancreatic regeneration. Amer. J. Path. **1**, 415 (1925).

— LECOMPTE, P. M.: The Pathology of Diabetes Mellitus. 3rd Ed. LEA and FEBIGER. Philadelphia 1952, p. 42.

WASSERMAN, P., BROH-KAHN, R. H., MIRSKY, I. A.: The antigenic property of insulin. J. Immunol. **38**, 213 (1940).

— MIRSKY, J. A.: Immunological identity of insulin from various species. Endokrin. **31**, 115 (1942).

WATTENWYL, N. VON, BÜRGI, H.: Morphologische Veränderungen der Langerhans'schen Inseln juveniler Ratten nach Behandlung mit Antiinsulin-Serum. Schweiz. med. Wschr. **24**, 314 (1964).

WAUGH, DIXON, CLAGETT, BOLLMAN, SPRAGUE, COMFORT (1946): cited by MARBLE (1959).

DE WECK, A., FREY, J. R.: Immunotolerance to simple chemicals. In: Monographs in Allergy, Vol. 1. p. Basel-New York: S. Karger 1966.

WEHNER, H., SCHADE, U., ASANTE, F.: Veränderungen an der glomerulären Basalmembran des Meerschweinchens durch Fremdinsulin und ihre Beziehung zur Höhe der Insulin-Bindungsfähigkeit des Serums. Virch. Arch. Abt. A Path. Anat. **348**, 164 (1969).

WEIGLE, W. O.: Autoimmunity and termination of acquired immunological tolerance. 3rd Intern. Symposium on Immunopathology. La Jolla. Basel: Benno Schwabe 1963, p. 167.

WELSH, G. W., HENLEY, E. D., WILLIAMS, R. H., COX, R. S.: J^{131}-Insulin metabolism in man. Plasma binding distribution and degradation. Amer. J. Med. **21**, 324 (1956).

WHITE, R. G.: Observations on the formation and nature of Russell bodies. Brit. J. exp. Path. **35**, 365 (1954).

— Functional recognition of immunologically competent cells by means of the fluorescent antibody technique. In: The immunologically competent cell. Ciba Found Study Group No. 16. Ed. by. G. W. WOLSTENHOLME and J. KNIGHT. London: Churchill 1963, p. 6.

WHITE, R. G., COONS, A. H., CONOLLY, J. M.: Studies on antibody-production. III. The alumn granuloma Studies on antibody production. IV. The role of a wax fraction of mycobacterium tuberculosis in adjuvant emulsions on the production of antibody to egg albumin. J. exp. Med. **102,** 73 (1955).

VAN DE WIEL, W. W. M., VAN DE WIEL-DORFMEYER, H.: Insulin antibodies (letter to the editor). Lancet **1964 I,** 561.

WILLIAMS, R. H., ELGEE, N. J., LEE, N. D., HOGNESS, J.-R., WONG, T.: Insulin metabolism. Trans. Ass. Amer. Physiol. **66,** 137 (1953).

WILSON, S.: The antigenic loci in insulin. Proc. 6th Int. Diab. Fed. Stockholm, 1967. Excerpta Medica Foundation. Ed.: J. ÖSTMAN. Amsterdam 1969, p. 403.

WITTEN, T. A., WANG, W. L., KILLIAN, M.: Reaction of lymphocytes with purified protein derivative conjugated with fluorescein. Science **142,** 596 (1963).

WRIGHT, P. H.: "Production on Acute Insulin Deficiency by Administration of Insulin Antiserum". Nature **183,** 829 (1959).

— Experimental insulin deficiency due to insulin antibodies. In: Handbuch des Diabetes mellitus. I. Hrsg.: E. F. PFEIFFER. München: J. F. Lehmanns Verlag 1969, p. 841.

— KRISBERG, R. A., HALPERN, B., DOLKART, R. E.: "Properties of insulin antibodies produced by the guinea-pig, horse, sheep, and man. Diabetes **11,** 519 (1962).

— NORMAN, L. L.: Some factors affecting insulin antibody production in guinea pigs. Diabetes **15,** 668 (1966).

— MAKULU, D. R.: Some immunological properties of insulin and proinsulin. Diabetes **18** (Suppl.) 339 (1969) Abstr.

YAGI, Y., MAIER, P., PRESSMAN, D.: Two different anti-insulin antibodies in guinea pig antisera. J. Immunol. **89,** 442 (1962).

— — — ARBESMAN, C. E., REISMAN, R. E., LENZNER, A. R.: Multiplicity of insulin binding antibodies in human sera". J. Immunol. **90,** 760 (1963).

YALOW, R. S., BERSON, S. A.: Assay of plasma insulin in human subjects by immunologic methods. Nature **184,** 1648 (1959).

ZEITZ, ST. V., ARSDEL, P. P. VAN, MCCLURE, D.: Specific response of human leucocytes to pollen antigen in tissue culture. J. Allergy **38,** 321 (1966).

ZIEGLER, M., LIPPMANN, H. G.: Gewinnung praecipitierender Insulin-Antikörper von der Ziege, Caper domesticus. Experientia (Basel) **25,** 191 (1969).

Subject Index

Monographs on Endocrinology

Already Published:

Vol. 1: Ohno, S., Sex Chromosomes and Sex-linked Genes. With 33 figures. X, 192 pages. 1967. DM 38,—

Vol. 2: Eik-Nes, K. B., and E. C. Horning, Gas Phase Chromatography of Steroids. With 85 figures. XV, 382 pages. 1968. DM 38,—

Vol. 3: Sulman, F. G., Hypothalamic Control of Lactation. With 58 figures. XII, 235 pages. 1970. DM 52,—

Vol. 4: Westphal, U., Steroid-Protein Interactions. With 144 figures. XIII, 567 pages. 1971. DM 86,—

Vol. 5: Müller, J., Regulation of Aldosterone Biosynthesis. With 19 figures. VII, 139 pages. 1971. DM 36,—

Vol. 6: Federlin, K., Immunopathology of Insulin. Clinical and Experimental Studies. With 53 figures. XIV, 185 pages. 1971. DM 49,60

In Preparation:

Baulieu, E. E., Bicêtre: Current Problems in the Metabolism of Steroid Hormones.

Berson, S. A./Yalow, R. S., New York: Immunoassay of Peptide Hormones.

Borth, R., Toronto: Clinical Hormone Assays.

Breuer, H./Rao, G. S., Bonn: Metabolism of Estrogens.

Caldeyro-Barcia, R., Montevideo: Oxytocin.

Copp, D. H., Vancouver: Calcitonin.

Edelman, I. S., San Francisco: Aldosterone: Gene Action and Sodium Transport.

Gregory, R. A., Liverpool/Grossman, M. I., Los Angeles: The Gastrins.

Gurpide, E., Minneapolis: Tracer Methods in Hormone Research.

Horton, W. E., London: Prostaglandins.

Jensen, E./Desombre, E., Chicago: Receptors and Action of Estradiol.

Lunenfeld, B., Tel Hashomer: Gonadotropins.

McKenzie, J. M., Montreal: The Pathogenesis of Graves' Disease.

Neumann/Steinbeck/Elger, Berlin: Hormones in Sexual Differentiation.

Renold, A. E./Stauffacher, W., Geneva: Pathophysiology of Diabetes.

Roberts, S., Los Angeles: Subcellular Mechanisms in the Regulation of Corticosteroidgenesis.

Short, R. V., Cambridge: The Ovary and its Hormones.

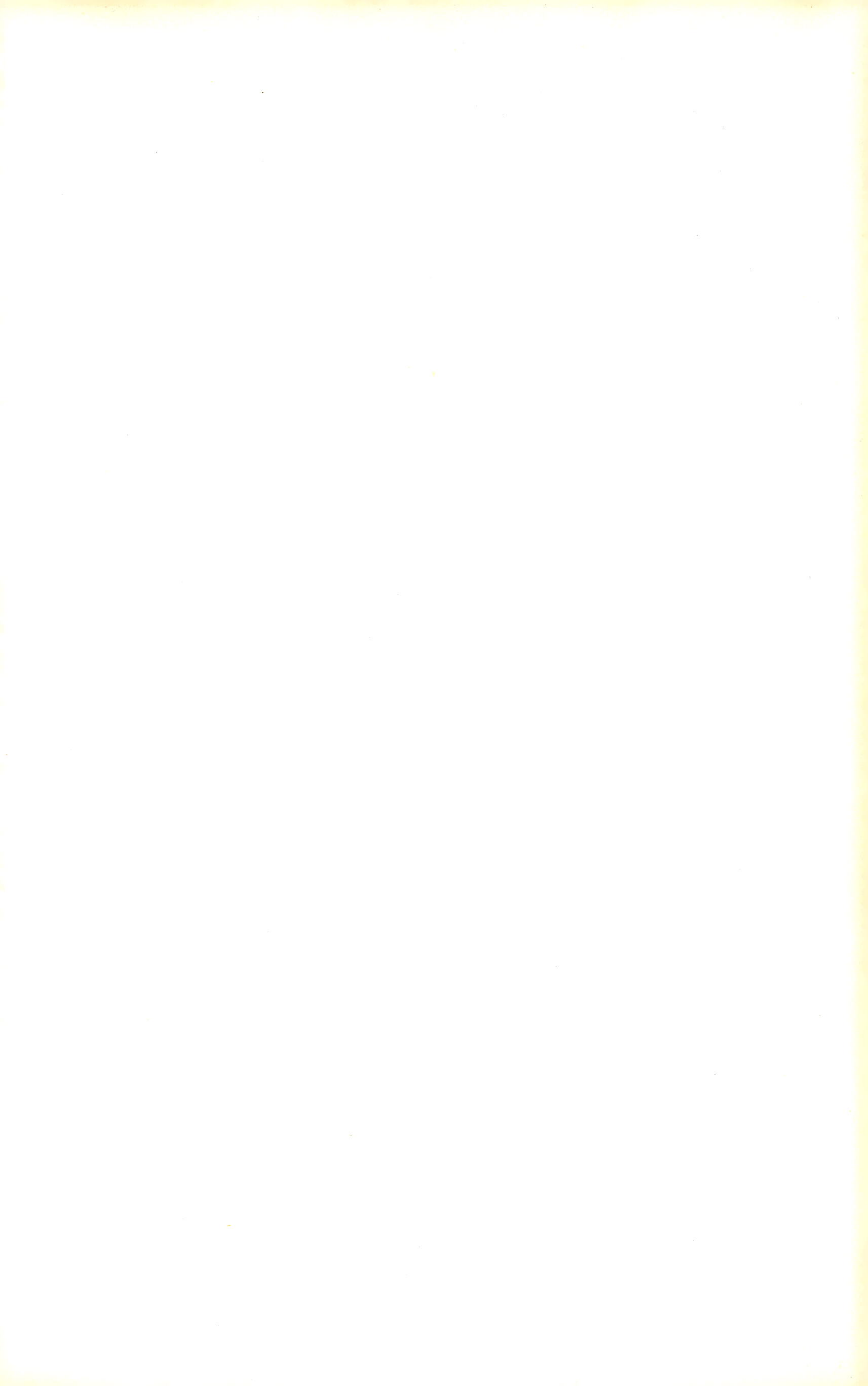